Get Through

Intercollegiate MRCS Parts 1 and 2: MCQs and EMQs

Get Through

Intercollegiate MRCS Parts 1 and 2: MCQs and EMQs

Simon Overstall MBBS MRCS

Senior House Officer in Plastic Surgery, St George's Hospital, London, UK

Giles Cunnick MBBS BSc MD FRCS

Consultant Breast and General Surgeon, High Wycombe, UK

Kefah Mokbel MBBS MS FRCS

Consultant Breast and General Surgeon, St George's Hospital, Professor of Cancer Genetics and Pharmacogenomics, Brunel Institute, London, UK

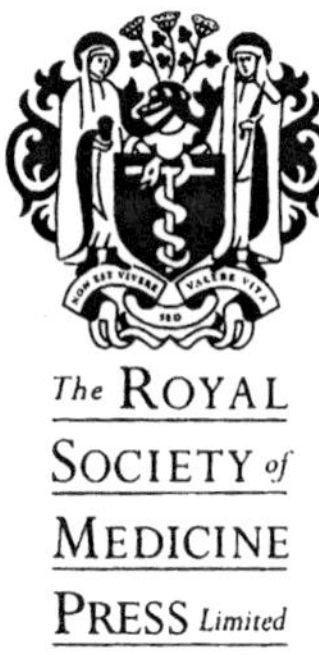

The ROYAL SOCIETY of MEDICINE PRESS Limited

Reprinted 2006, 2009

Published by the Royal Society of Medicine Press Ltd
1 Wimpole Street, London W1G 0AE, UK
Tel: +44 (0)20 7290 2921
Fax: +44 (0)20 7290 2929
E-mail: publishing@rsm.ac.uk
Website: www.rsmpress.co.uk

British Library Cataloguing in Publication Data
A catalogue record for this book is available from the British Library

ISBN: 1-85315-595-0

Distribution in Europe and Rest of the World:

Marston Book Services Ltd
PO Box 269
Abingdon
Oxon OX14 4YN, UK
Tel: +44 (0)1235 465500
Fax: +44 (0)1235 465666

Distribution in USA and Canada:

Royal Society of Medicine Press Ltd
c/o JAMCO Distribution Inc
1401 Lakeway Drive
Lewisville, TX 75057, USA
Tel: +1 800 538 1287
Fax: +1 972 353 1303
E-mail: jamco@majors.com

Distribution in Australia and New Zealand:

Elsevier Australia
30–52 Smidmore Street
Marrikville NSW 2204, Australia
Tel: +61 2 9517 8999
Fax: +61 2 9517 2249
E-mail: service@elsevier.com.au

Typeset by S R Nova Pvt Ltd, Bangalore, India
Printed in the UK by Bell & Bain Ltd, Glasgow

Contents

Preface

The format of the MRCS examinations changed in January 2004. The intercollegiate exam was introduced to replace the previously separate papers of the Royal Colleges of Surgeons of England, Edinburgh, Glasgow and Ireland.

The old style 'core' and 'systems' papers have now been replaced with Paper 1 (multiple choice questions in applied basic science) and Paper 2 (extended matching questions in clinical problem solving). The two exams are held on the same day. Most candidates sit both papers at the same time, although it is possible to sit them separately. To be eligible for the exams, the candidate must be in a recognized surgical training post.

After successfully passing both written papers and after completing four recognized SHO posts, the candidate is eligible to sit the viva and clinical exams in order to become a member of one of the Royal Colleges of Surgeons.

This book is designed to help those candidates who are about to sit the first two parts of the MRCS exam. There is no better way to prepare for an MCQ exam than by practising with hundreds of MCQ papers beforehand. The style of and difficulty of the questions in this book are designed to be similar to the actual exam in order to make the experience as realistic as possible. Indeed, many of the questions are based on actual exam questions that previous candidates have remembered. You will notice that certain topics are repeated throughout this book. Take this as a hint that they are topics worth learning! This book is designed as an adjunct to be used with other revision texts. The papers should be attempted after working through a good surgical textbook and relevant journals in order to test understanding as well as to highlight gaps in your knowledge.

Set yourself the allocated time and treat these papers as mock exams. The pass mark for the exams varies from time to time, but is around 75%. Unlike many medical student exams, the MRCS papers have no negative marking. If you don't know the answer, it is a good idea to guess (for the MCQs you have a 50% chance of getting it right). No answers should be left blank.

It cannot be overemphasized how important it is to read the question carefully before answering. Under the stress of the exam and in the perceived lack of time, it is all too easy to skim through the questions and miss vital clues. Relax. Go slowly. You do actually have plenty of time. Read the question fully. Stop. Think. Then answer.

Finally, even though this book is designed for candidates sitting the MRCS exam, much of the subject matter is very similar to surgical finals, although in greater depth. This book is therefore eminently suited to brighter medical students looking for prizes or those with an interest in surgery as a future career.

Good luck!

Simon Overstall
Giles Cunnick
Kefah Mokbel

Practice Paper I

Applied Basic Sciences – MCQs

- This paper consists of 90 multiple true/false questions.
- Each question contains a variable number of items.
- Each item may be true or false.
- It is possible for the items in any one question to be all true, all false or any intermediate combination.
- Because of the variable number of items, a mark will not necessarily be required for every part of the answer sheet.
- Marks will not be deducted for a wrong answer. Equally, you will not gain a mark if you mark both true and false.
- Only answers that are clearly struck horizontally across the correct response will guarantee a mark.
- Faint marking may be misread. All scores within 5 marks of the pass mark will be scrutinized.

Practice Paper 1: Part 1 – MCQs in Applied Basic Sciences

1. **The following are Gram-positive organisms:**

   A Group A *Streptococcus*
   B MRSA
   C *Neisseria gonorrhoeae*
   D *Clostridium tetani*
   E *Klebsiella*

2. **The following statements are true regarding exotoxins:**

   A The lipopolysaccharide portion of the cell wall of Gram-negative bacteria is an example of an exotoxin.
   B Most are polypeptides.
   C Tetanus toxoid is an example of an exotoxin.
   D Botulinum toxin is an example of an exotoxin.
   E Exotoxins are usually more heat-labile than endotoxins.

3. **The following criteria should be met in order to diagnose brain stem death:**

   A fixed and unresponsive pupils
   B absent pulse
   C absent spontaneous respiration when $PaCO_2 > 6.65\,\text{kPa}$
   D absent gag reflex
   E absent spinal reflexes

4. **The following diseases are caused by *Clostridia* spp.:**

   A tetanus
   B pseudomembranous colitis
   C gas gangrene
   D anthrax
   E botulism food poisoning

5. **The brachial plexus**

   A The long thoracic nerve receives fibres from C5, C6, C7, C8 and T1.
   B The posterior cord of the brachial plexus divides into the radial and axillary nerves.
   C The median nerve is a branch of both the medial and the lateral cords.
   D The long thoracic nerve supplies the latissimus dorsi muscle.
   E Branches of the posterior cord of the brachial plexus supply the muscles of the posterior wall of the axilla.

6. **Pleomorphic adenoma of the parotid**

A has a true capsule
B is treated with radiotherapy alone in most cases
C does not recur after surgical removal
D is the most common tumour of the parotid
E is a recognized cause of facial nerve palsy

7. **The shoulder**

A The quadrangular space is bounded by the teres major muscle superiorly and the teres minor muscle inferiorly.
B Anterior dislocation of the shoulder may lead to avulsion of the inferior glenohumeral ligament.
C The subscapularis tendon inserts into the greater tuberosity of the humerus.
D The accessory nerve is at risk of damage in humeral neck fractures.
E Fractures of the humerus rarely need surgical intervention.

8. **The following structures pass through the carpal tunnel:**

A median nerve
B radial artery
C flexor policis longus (FPL) tendon
D all the flexor digitorum profundus (FDP) tendons
E flexor carpi radialis (FCR) tendon

9. **In the systemic inflammatory response syndrome (SIRS)**

A causes may include peritonitis, burns and haemorrhage
B insulin release is reduced
C the white count may be elevated above 12 or reduced below 4 as one of the diagnostic criteria
D a metabolic alkalosis may develop
E nitrous oxide may be used for treatment of vasoconstriction

10. **The intra-aortic balloon pump (IABP)**

A is contraindicated in severe aortic regurgitation
B increases blood pressure by increasing total peripheral resistance (TPR)
C is inflated in diastole and deflated in systole
D is useful in septic shock
E increases the mean arterial pressure (MAP)

11. Epistaxis

A Bleeding is usually from Little's area on the lateral nasal wall.
B Pressure over the bony root of the nose is a useful technique to slow the bleeding.
C A visible bleeding area may be successfully cauterized with a silver nitrate stick.
D Bleeding from a site not visible may be treated by packing the nasal cavity with cocaine-soaked ribbon gauze.
E Ligation of the internal carotid artery may be necessary in torrential bleeding that does not respond to simple measures.

12. The scaphoid bone

A articulates with the 1st metacarpal
B is palpable in the anatomical snuff-box
C articulates with the lunate
D receives its blood supply from a distal origin
E provides attachment for the flexor retinaculum

13. Hypercalcaemia can be caused by

A malignancy
B osteoporosis
C Paget's disease
D secondary hyperparathyroidism
E pancreatitis

14. Adult respiratory distress syndrome (ARDS)

A can be caused by burns
B can be caused by heart failure
C has characteristic chest X-ray appearances
D has a low associated morbidity
E may form part of the systemic inflammatory response syndrome

15. The epiploic foramen

A is bound anteriorly by the free edge of the greater omentum
B is situated posterior to the common bile duct
C lies inferior to the caudate surface of the liver
D is an important landmark for the 'Pringle manoeuvre'
E allows communication between the greater and lesser sacs

16. Which of the following surgical techniques lead to improved wound healing?

A atraumatic handling of tissue
B tension-less wound edge apposition
C approximation of underlying fatty tissue to obliterate dead space
D protecting the wound from water for at least one week
E meticulous haemostasis

17. **Which of the following are associated with arterial or venous thrombosis and embolic phenomenon?**

A factor V Leiden mutation
B heparin-associated thrombocytopenia
C antithrombin III deficiency
D von Willebrand's disease
E vitamin C deficiency

18. **Which of the following factors decreases collagen synthesis, thereby delaying wound healing?**

A malnutrition
B infection
C anaemia
D advanced age
E hypoxia

19. **Which of the following factors influences cerebral blood flow?**

A arterial pCO_2
B arterial pO_2
C systemic arterial blood pressure
D preoperative neurological dysfunction
E intracranial pressure

20. **Local anaesthetics**

A work best in their ionized form
B inhibit transmission of nerve impulses by increasing sodium membrane permeability
C are classified as either amides or esters
D produce peripheral vasodilation
E are weak acids

21. **Which of the following statements regarding hypercalcaemia are true?**

A The symptoms of hypercalcaemia may mimic some symptoms of hyperglycaemia.
B Metastatic breast cancer is an unusual cause of hypercalcaemia.
C Calcitonin is a satisfactory long-term therapy for hypercalcaemia.
D Severely hypercalcaemic patients exhibit the signs of extracellular fluid volume deficit.
E Urinary calcium excretion may be increased by vigorous volume repletion.

22. **Which of the following statements about thyroid follicular carcinoma are true?**

A It usually presents at an earlier age than papillary carcinoma.
B It disseminates via haematogenous routes.
C It is the most common type of well-differentiated thyroid carcinoma.
D It metastasizes to bone.
E Follicular carcinomas are frequently multicentric.

23. **Thyroid physiology**

A The iodine utilized in hormone synthesis is derived principally from dietary sources.
B The role of thyroid-stimulating hormone (TSH) is limited to regulation of the release of thyroid hormone.
C Enough thyroxine (T_4) is stored in the normal thyroid to provide a euthyroid state for 3 weeks despite absence of iodine intake.
D The regulation of thyroid function involves pituitary but not hypothalamic input.
E Mono-iodothyronine is combined with di-iodothyronine to produce tri-iodothyronine (T_3).

24. **Which of the following conditions of the adrenal gland are usually treated medically?**

A Conn syndrome
B Adrenocortical carcinoma
C Congenital adrenal hyperplasia
D Cushing's disease
E Phaeochromocytoma

25. **The parathyroid glands**

A develop from the second and third pharyngeal pouches, along with the palatine tonsil and the thymus
B migrate caudally in the neck in normal development but can be found anywhere from the pharyngeal mucosa to the deep mediastinum
C secrete PTH and calcitonin to manage calcium homeostasis
D usually number four, but only number two or three in 20% of the population
E contain enzymes that catalyse the conversion of 25-hydroxyvitamin D_3 to 1,25-dihydroxyvitamin D_3

26. **Which of the following are not components of the multiple endocrine neoplasia (MEN) type 2B syndrome?**

    A multiple neuromas on the lips, tongue and oral mucosa
    B hyperparathyroidism
    C medullary thyroid cancer
    D phaeochromocytoma
    E pituitary adenomas

27. **Hyperthyroidism can be caused by which of the following conditions?**

    A Graves' disease
    B Plummer's disease
    C iatrogenic thyroxine administration
    D Hashimoto's disease
    E medullary carcinoma of the thyroid

28. **Common causes of goitrous hypothyroidism in adults are**

    A Graves' disease
    B Riedel's thyroiditis
    C Hashimoto's disease
    D de Quervain's thyroiditis
    E multinodular goitre

29. **Which of the following statements about head injuries are true?**

    A The majority of deaths from road traffic accidents are due to head injuries.
    B Head injury alone often produces shock.
    C A rapid neurological examination is part of the initial evaluation of the trauma patient.
    D Optimizing oxygenation of the brain is part of initial therapy.
    E Dilated pupils may be due to opiate administration.

30. **Which of the following tumours may cause elevated levels of carcino-embryonic antigen (CEA)?**

    A breast cancer
    B colorectal cancer
    C gastric cancer
    D lung cancer
    E testicular cancer

31. **The presence of which of the following indicates a poor prognosis for patients with breast cancer?**

    A CEA
    B c-*erb*B-2
    C AFP
    D Human chorionic gonadotrophin (hCG)
    E oestrogen receptors

32. **Which of the following statements regarding the inherited form of retinoblastoma are correct?**

A Retinoblastoma results from amplification of the H-*ras* oncogene.
B Clinical disease results after chromosomal loss in a retinal cell after birth.
C Retinoblastoma results from the loss of a tumour suppressor gene.
D Clinical disease results from a chromosomal translocation.
E The overall mortality rate is approximately 10%.

33. **For which of the following tumours have DNA viruses been implicated as aetiological agents?**

A Burkitt lymphoma
B testicular carcinoma
C cervical carcinoma
D hepatocellular carcinoma
E oesophageal carcinoma

34. **In a patient who has chronic, complete occlusion of a common iliac artery, which of the following are true?**

A Symptoms are usually claudication of the calf muscles only.
B Symptoms are usually claudication of the thigh and calf.
C The decision whether or not to operate can be based on clinical examination findings.
D Collateral iliac arterial vessels are usually patent.
E Balloon angioplasty is appropriate in some patients.

35. **The hepatic artery**

A supplies the same amount of blood to the liver as the portal vein
B provides the same amount of oxygen to the liver as the portal vein
C contains blood with the same oxygenation as the portal vein
D supplies most of the blood to hepatic metastases
E divides the liver into anatomical segments

36. **Diathermy**

A Accidental burns are most commonly caused by incorrect application of the patient plate.
B Diathermy should not be used in its monopolar form on the testis.
C It should be avoided with pacemakers, if possible.
D Current follows the pathway of minimal resistance.
E Patient plates should be placed as far from the operating field as possible.

37. **Sodium homeostasis**

A The most common cause of hyponatraemia is a deficit in total body sodium.
B Hypernatraemia is usually the result of excessive sodium administration.
C Most surgical patients with hyponatraemia are best treated by free-water restriction.
D Central nervous system effects are the predominant symptom of hypernatraemia.
E Hypernatraemia should be rapidly corrected with free-water administration.

38. **The testes**

A The testicular artery arises from the internal iliac artery.
B The right testicular vein usually enters the right renal vein.
C The Leydig cells produce testosterone.
D Each primary spermatocyte gives rise to four spermatozoa.
E A patent processus vaginalis predisposes to direct inguinal hernia formation.

39. **The following are potential complications of benign prostatic hyperplasia:**

A urinary calculi
B bladder diverticulae
C prostate cancer development
D renal failure
E urinary infections

40. **The following structures form the anterior part of the rectus sheath below the arcuate line:**

A external oblique aponeurosis
B internal oblique aponeurosis
C tranversus abdominis aponeurosis
D transversalis fascia
E Scarpa's fascia

41. **The following features differentiate the large bowel from the small bowel:**

A haustrations
B taeniae coli
C appendices epiploicae
D longitudinal peristalsis
E mesentery

42. **Osteogenic sarcoma**

A has two age peaks of incidence
B when affecting the limb, is treated by amputation in most cases
C has X-ray features including 'Codman's triangle'
D most commonly affects the metaphysis of the femur
E develops in a third of patients with Paget's disease of the bone

43. **The following structures are retroperitoneal:**

A stomach
B spleen
C second part of the duodenum
D all of the pancreas
E descending colon

44. **When the renin–angiotensin–aldosterone system is stimulated by hypovolaemia**

A renin converts angiotensin I to angiotensin II
B angiotensin II causes vasoconstriction of the efferent glomerular arteriole
C angiotensin II stimulates the adrenal medulla to synthesize aldosterone
D angiotensin II stimulates the adrenal cortex to increase cortisol production
E angiotensin-converting enzymes degrade bradykinin

45. **The transpyloric plane**

A is halfway between the suprasternal notch and the symphysis pubis
B corresponds to the level of L1
C is the level at which the aorta gives off the superior mesenteric artery
D is the level at which the spinal cord terminates
E corresponds to the level at which the lateral border of the rectus crosses the costal margin

46. **Carcinoma of the pancreas**

A is more common in men
B has its peak incidence in patients aged 60–80
C is more common in smokers
D has a 5-year survival rate of approximately 30%
E is usually treated surgically

47. **Carcinoma of the oesophagus**

A It is more common in men.
B It is more common in patients with Plummer–Vinson syndrome.
C In western countries, adenocarcinoma is three times more common than squamous cell carcinoma.
D Ivor–Lewis oesophagectomy is suitable for upper-third tumours.
E The 5-year survival rate is approximately 20%.

48. **The following tumours commonly metastasize to bone:**

A gastric
B bronchus
C breast
D testicular
E osteosarcoma

49. **Melanoma**

A The incidence is increasing.
B The superficial spreading type is the most common.
C Breslow thickness and the presence of ulceration affect prognosis.
D Sentinel node biopsy has been shown to be an effective treatment.
E Melanomas on the trunk carry a better prognosis than those on the limbs.

50. **Thyroid cancer**

A It is more common in men.
B It is associated with previous exposure to radiation.
C It is most commonly a follicular tumour.
D Anaplastic carcinomas carry the worst prognosis.
E It may form part of the MEN type 1 syndrome.

51. **Thyroid cancer**

A Serum calcitonin is a useful marker for medullary cancers.
B It is usually treated by thyroid lobectomy.
C Radioactive iodine can be used in the treatment of follicular carcinomas.
D Papillary carcinomas may be associated with parathyroid adenomas and phaeochromocytomas.
E It may present with a change in the voice.

52. **Lung cancer**

A It is the most common cancer in the UK.
B It is most commonly of the small cell type.
C It may present with neurological changes in the hand.
D Squamous cell tumours have the worst prognosis.
E Adenocarcinomas are most common in smokers.

53. **The following are risk factors for lung cancer:**

A asbestos
B passive smoking
C radon gas
D tuberculosis
E chronic obstructive pulmonary disease

54. **Prostate cancer**

A has a high incidence in American Afro-Caribbeans
B most commonly arises in the central zone
C commonly metastasizes to bone to cause a lytic lesion
D is usually of the adenocarcinoma cell type
E is suggested by a PSA of 20 ng/ml

55. **Pancreatitis**

A in western countries is most commonly due to either gallstones or alcohol
B may be iatrogenic
C may cause hypercalcaemia
D is usually managed by the surgical team, as most patients eventually need operative treatment
E has a poorer prognosis in the presence of hyperlipidaemia

56. **Ranson's criteria give a score for each of the following:**

A age over 65
B amylase over 1000 iu/l
C glucose over 11.2 mmol/l
D calcium over 2 mmol/l
E white blood cell count over 16

57. **Phaeochromocytoma**

A is a tumour arising from the chromaffin cells of the adrenal medulla
B is a tumour in which 20% of cases are malignant
C may be detected by measuring urinary levels of 5-HIAA
D may arise from outside the adrenals
E may form part of the MEN type 1 syndrome

58. **Bowel polyps**

A Metaplastic (hyperplastic) polyps have a propensity for malignant transformation.
B Hamartomatous polyps may be associated with periorbital pigmentation.
C May lead to microcytic anaemia.
D Tubular adenomas are more prone to malignant transformation than villous adenomas.
E Intestinal hamartomas are a feature of the Osler–Weber–Rendu syndrome.

59. **Familial adenosis polyposis**

A is an autosomal recessive disease
B is associated with a gene carried on the short arm of chromosome 15
C tends to first affect patients in their 60s and 70s
D rarely needs surgical intervention nowadays
E may be associated with epidermoid cysts

60. **Breast surgery**

A 50% of breast cancer cases are hereditary.
B Centrally located tumours are usually amenable to wide local excision.
C Tamoxifen is only indicated in hormone receptor-positive patients.
D Axillary node clearance is indicated in a patient with 1 cm^3 volume of DCIS.
E Radiotherapy is rarely necessary after adequate wide local excision.

61. **Peptic ulceration**

A *Helicobacter pylori* infection has an important aetiological role.
B Peptic ulceration is more commonly treated by surgical intervention nowadays.
C It is more common in developing countries.
D It is more common in smokers.
E It can be associated with pancreatic tumours.

62. ***Helicobacter pylori***

A is a Gram-positive organism
B is a micro-aerophilic, spiral-shaped organism
C infection causes an increase in gastric acid production
D produces urease enzyme that helps to lower the surrounding pH
E is most commonly treated with 'double therapy': a proton pump inhibitor and an antibiotic

63. **The following plasma hormone levels increase following trauma:**

A aldosterone
B testosterone
C growth hormone
D cortisol
E noradrenaline

64. **Atherosclerosis**

A is named after the Greek for 'hard porridge'
B is another name for cholesterol deposits on the surface of the intima
C rarely causes thrombosis unless the plaque ruptures
D may cause erectile dysfunction
E is the most common cause of upper-limb ischaemia

65. **'Reducible' risk factors for peripheral vascular disease include**

A smoking
B diabetes
C male sex
D hypertension
E HRT

66. **Thoracic aortic dissection**

A of type A only affects the aorta proximal to the left subclavian artery
B of type B has a similar outcome when managed medically or surgically
C can be a cause of aortic valve regurgitation
D may cause ECG changes mimicking a myocardial infarction
E is more common in males

67. **Renal and ureteric calculi**

A are more common in surgeons than the general public
B are most commonly 'triple phosphate' stones
C are associated with inflammatory bowel disease
D predispose to transitional cell tumour formation
E usually require surgical intervention

68. The incidence of gallstones is increased by the following conditions:

A obesity
B liver cirrhosis
C thalassaemia
D inflammatory bowel disease
E viral hepatitis

69. The following are DNA viruses:

A herpesvirus
B influenza virus
C measles virus
D human papillomavirus
E HIV

70. Iron deficiency

A causes a macrocytic anaemia
B is associated with spoon-shaped nails
C is associated with dysphagia
D causes a painful glossitis
E is more common in women

71. The following are typical of Crohn's disease:

A 'skip' lesions
B mucosal 'pseudopolyps'
C deep fissures and ulcers
D non-caseating epitheloid granulomas
E disease usually limited to the mucosa

72. General considerations in surgery

A Hair around the operative site is best shaved the day before surgery.
B Bathing in chlorhexidine prior to surgery has been shown to reduce the risk of wound infection.
C MRSA-positive patients should be placed at the start of the operating list, as they are usually the sickest patients.
D Surgical masks have been shown to reduce the risk of wound infection.
E Steroids impair wound healing, so should be stopped immediately preoperatively.

73. **Wound infections and surgery**

A Appendicectomy for appendicitis is a 'clean-contaminated' wound.
B An open fracture is a 'contaminated' wound.
C An uncomplicated inguinal hernia repair is a 'clean' wound.
D An elective uncomplicated right hemicolectomy is a 'dirty' wound.
E Hartmann's procedure for perforated diverticulitis is a 'contaminated' wound.

74. **Arterial blood pressure**

A The arterial pressure is proportional to cardiac output divided by systemic vascular resistance.
B The mean arterial pressure is halfway between the diastolic and systolic pressures.
C The dichrotic notch corresponds to opening of the aortic valve.
D Arterial pressure is monitored by baroreceptors in the carotid bodies.
E It is a reliable measurement of hypovolaemia.

75. **The cardiac cycle**

A The first heart sound corresponds to opening of the mitral and tricuspid valves.
B The QRS complex corresponds to the start of systole.
C The prolonged refractory period of the cardiac myocyte action potential is due to the opening of 'slow' potassium ion channels.
D The a-wave of the jugular venous waveform corresponds to closure of the aortic valve.
E The A–V node rapidly conducts the action potential from the atria to the ventricles.

76. **The anterior pituitary gland secretes the following hormones:**

A prolactin
B oxytocin
C thyroxine
D gonadotrophin-releasing hormone (GnRH)
E adrenocorticotrophic hormone (ACTH)

77. **Renal physiology**

A Normal glomerular filtration rate (GFR) is approximately 125 litres/min.
B Most sodium reabsorption occurs in the loop of Henle.
C The ascending limb of the loop of Henle is impervious to water.
D Antidiuretic hormone (ADH) increases the water permeability of the collecting ducts.
E Aldosterone increases potassium secretion in the distal convoluted tubule.

78. **Lung volumes**

A The vital capacity is equal to the inspiratory reserve volume plus the expiratory reserve volume.
B The minute volume is equal to the respiratory rate times the tidal volume.
C Total lung capacity is easily measured using spirometry.
D An FEV1/FVC ratio of less than 0.7 implies a restrictive lung defect.
E The residual volume is the same as the dead space.

79. **Haemoglobin physiology**

A Haemoglobin consists of an Fe-containing porphyrin ring with five globin polypeptides.
B The oxygen dissociation curve has a sigmoid shape.
C A rise in pCO_2 shifts the oxygen dissociation curve to the right.
D A rise in pH shifts the oxygen dissociation curve to the left.
E Each gram of haemoglobin can bind approximately 1.34 ml of oxygen.

80. **Vitamin D physiology**

A 25-Hydroxyvitamin D is converted to 1,25-dihydroxyvitamin D in the liver.
B Vitamin D is obtained from the diet and also made in the skin.
C Parathyroid hormone (PTH) increases the production of 1,25-dihydroxyvitamin D.
D Vitamin D increases calcium secretion in the intestine.
E A lack of vitamin D may lead to rickets or osteomalacia.

81. **Menstrual cycle**

A The average cycle lasts approximately 28 days.
B The luteal phase corresponds to higher levels of progesterone.
C Ovulation is triggered by an FSH surge.
D Menstruation occurs at the end of the follicular phase.
E The corpus luteum secretes oestrogen and progesterone.

82. **Muscle physiology**

A The Golgi tendon apparatus is responsible for the knee jerk reflex.
B The thick filaments contain myosin, the thin filaments contain actin.
C The neurotransmitter at the neuromuscular junction is acetylcholine.
D Muscle contraction is calcium-dependent.
E The knee jerk reflex has to cross two synapses.

83. **Cervical spine X-rays**

A Such X-rays should be taken in a multiple-trauma patient.
B Swimmer's view allows assessment of upper cervical vertebrae.
C The whole of the vertebral body of T1 should be visible.
D These X-rays usually show a 6 mm atlanto-odontoid gap in adults.
E If they show a displacement of more than 50% of vertebral width, this usually indicates bilateral facet dislocation.

84. **The scalenus anterior muscle**

A attaches into the anterior tubercles of the transverse processes of the C1–C7 vertebrae
B attaches to the scalene tubercle of the 1st rib
C has the subclavian vein passing posterior to it
D has the subclavian artery passing anterior to it
E Lies deep to the prevertebral layer of deep cervical fascia

85. **The carotid artery**

A The carotid artery lies anterior to the prevertebral fascia.
B It has the sympathetic chain as an anterior relation.
C The external carotid artery has no branches within the neck.
D The carotid artery has an important function in blood pressure homeostasis.
E The external carotid artery divides into the superficial temporal and maxillary arteries as its terminal branches.

86. **The thyroid gland**

A The thyroid gland lies deep to the pre-tracheal layer of deep cervical fascia.
B It has a central isthmus at the level of the thyroid cartilage.
C The inferior thyroid artery is a branch of the carotid artery.
D The recurrent laryngeal nerve is at risk during ligation of the superior thyroid artery.
E The thyroid gland has a blood supply directly from the arch of the aorta in 10% of people.

87. Hyperacute renal transplant rejection

A is cell-mediated
B usually occurs within hours of transplantation
C does not respond to corticosteroids
D is best treated by removal of the transplant
E has an incidence that is decreased by the use of cyclosporin A

88. Compartments of the leg

A The tibialis anterior, flexor digitorum longus and flexor hallucis longus all run in the anterior compartment.
B The lateral compartment of the leg is supplied by the deep peroneal nerve.
C Damage to the tibial nerve leads to foot drop.
D The peroneus longus inserts into the lateral side of the foot.
E Fractures of the proximal fibular can lead to paralysis of the anterior and lateral muscle compartments.

89. The following structures pass through the jugular foramen:

A vagus nerve
B glossopharyngeal nerve
C hypoglossal nerve
D accessory nerve
E facial nerve

90. The latissimus dorsi muscle

A is supplied by the long thoracic nerve
B inserts into the floor of the bicipital groove of the humerus
C is an important muscle for rock-climbers
D derives its blood supply from the first part of the subclavian artery
E has a nerve supply arising from the posterior cord of the brachial plexus

Practice Paper 2: Part I – MCQs in Applied Basic Sciences

1. The following are recognized causes of mycotic aneurysms:

   A *Mycobacterium tuberculosis*
   B *Salmonella*
   C *Escherichia coli*
   D Marfan syndrome
   E *Staphylococcus aureus*

2. Buerger's disease

   A has an equal sex distribution
   B causes foot claudication
   C is a panarteritis
   D is more likely in older patients
   E will stabilize if the patient stops smoking

3. Dissecting aortic aneurysms

   A usually arise because of cystic medial necrosis
   B are usually accompanied by ECG changes suggestive of myocardial infarction
   C start in the ascending aorta in most cases
   D have an increased incidence in Marfan syndrome
   E are associated with hypertension

4. Torsion of the testicle

   A if it truly persists for more than 12 hours, has a high likelihood of irreversible ischaemia
   B may be initiated by trauma
   C is predisposed by having a bell-clapper testis
   D is much less common after age 25
   E may be diagnosed by colour flow Doppler

5. Treatments for pseudo-obstruction include

   A octreotide
   B colonoscopic decompression
   C nasogastric tube insertion
   D correction of hypokalaemia
   E caecostomy

6. **Bladder irrigation during a TURP may produce**

A haemolysis
B hyponatraemia
C haemodilution
D hypercalcaemia
E hyperkalaemia

7. **Childhood inguinal hernias are**

A more common in boys
B a known cause of testicular atrophy
C repaired only if they persist after the age of 5 years
D treated by simple herniotomy without mesh
E more common in premature-born children

8. **The following viruses are spread by the faecal–oral route:**

A hepatitis A
B hepatitis B
C hepatitis C
D hepatitis D
E hepatitis E

9. **Rhabdomyolysis may be caused by**

A compartment syndrome
B burns
C amphetamines
D *Salmonella*
E prolonged immobilization

10. **Acute mediastinitis**

A has a low mortality
B may occur after forceful vomiting
C often results in a marked tachycardia
D is not associated with chest X-ray changes
E may occur after upper GI endoscopy

11. **Burns**

A are responsible for 700–800 deaths per year in the UK
B result in a decrease in the metabolic rate
C are associated with a decrease in cardiac output
D cause a decrease in lung compliance in inhalational injuries
E to the chest do not require escharotomy

12. **The rotator cuff of the shoulder joint is formed by which of the following muscles?**

A subscapularis
B teres major
C pectoralis major
D deltoid
E infraspinatus

13. **Complications of tibial fractures include**

A leg shortening
B compartment syndrome
C delayed union
D tibial nerve damage
E fat embolism

14. **Avascular necrosis is particularly associated with fracture of the following bones:**

A third metacarpal
B scaphoid
C talus
D mandibular condyle
E neck of femur

15. **Gas embolism is a recognized complication of**

A varicose vein surgery
B criminal abortion
C blood transfusion
D deep-sea diving
E laparoscopic surgery

16. **The oesophagus**

A It is constricted by the left main bronchus.
B It is a site for portal–systemic anastomosis at its lower third.
C Lower-third lymphatic drainage ends in the coeliac lymph nodes.
D The upper third is the commonest site for oesophageal carcinoma.
E The thoracic part lies anterior to the left recurrent laryngeal nerve.

17. **The femoral triangle**

A The medial border is formed by the lateral border of the adductor longus.
B The lateral border is formed by the lateral border of the sartorius.
C The triangle contains the iliacus, psoas and pectineus in its floor.
D It contains the posterior division of the obturator nerve.
E It has a gutter-shaped floor.

18. **The following are correct statements regarding lung volumes:**

 A Tidal volume is approximately 0.5 litres in an average person.
 B Tidal volume + functional residual capacity = expiratory reserve volume.
 C Inspiratory reserve volume + tidal volume + residual volume = vital capacity.
 D Vital capacity + residual volume = total lung capacity.
 E Residual capacity is the volume of air remaining in the lung after a maximal expiration.

19. **Recognized complications of aortic aneurysm repair include**

 A trash foot
 B ischaemic colitis
 C graft infection
 D paraplegia
 E incisional hernia

20. **The differential diagnosis of a groin lump in a supine patient may include**

 A torsion of the testicle
 B psoas abscess
 C Hodgkin lymphoma
 D saphena varix
 E spigelian hernia

21. **The following sutures are usually absorbed within 4 months:**

 A polyglycolic acid (Dexon)
 B polydioxanone (PDS)
 C silk
 D Polyamide (nylon)
 E Polygalactic acid (Vicryl)

22. **The following may cause a fall in the platelet count in peripheral blood:**

 A DIC
 B massive transfusion
 C aspirin
 D warfarin
 E heparin

23. **Pulse oximetry**

A It is based on Beer's law.
B It has a mean error of less than 5%.
C Readings are not affected in carbon monoxide poisoning.
D Readings are not affected by nail polish when using finger probes.
E It usually uses six wavelengths of light.

24. **Grade III haemorrhagic shock**

A It occurs after the sudden loss of 1.5–2.0 litres of blood.
B It is associated with a narrowed pulse pressure.
C It is associated with a near normal heart rate.
D The systolic blood pressure is normal.
E The respiratory rate is usually elevated to >20 breaths/min.

25. **The hand**

A The flexor digitorum profundus (FDP) inserts into the distal phalynx of the digits.
B The lumbricals arise from the flexor digitorum superficialis (FDS) tendon and insert into the dorsal extensor expansion.
C The lumbricals run across the ulnar aspect of the corresponding metacarpal–phalangeal joint (MCPJ).
D All intrinsic muscles of the hand are supplied by T1.
E All intrinsic muscles of the hand are supplied by the ulnar nerve.

26. **The following deaths require a postmortem by the coroner:**

A death within 24 hours of any operation
B death following accidental administration of the wrong drug dose
C death due to metastatic disease during chemotherapy
D death following chest drain insertion for a chronic effusion
E death following nasogastric tube insertion in a patient with a GCS of 14, and mastoid bruising following a head injury

27. **Ulnar nerve injury at the wrist causes**

A clawhand
B wasting of the second lumbrical muscle
C wasting of the thenar eminence
D weakness of wrist extension
E sensory impairment over the medial one and a half fingers

28. **The following stimulate renin release:**

A a rise in blood pressure
B propranolol
C salt depletion
D angiotensin II
E an increase in plasma K^+ concentration

29. **Necrotizing enterocolitis:**

A is associated with redcurrant jelly stools, which are pathognomonic of the condition
B typically occurs in children between 3 months and 2 years of age
C is often fatal
D presents with abdominal distension, vomiting and diarrhoea
E is often primarily caused by *Salmonella*

30. **Portosystemic anastomoses occur**

A around the appendix
B at the bare area of the liver
C at the lower end of the rectum
D around the umbilicus
E at the lower third of the oesophagus

31. **Medical causes of acute abdominal pain include**

A right lower lobe pneumonia
B lead poisoning
C hepatitis
D porphyria
E diabetic ketoacidosis

32. **The following are well-recognized associations with right upper quadrant pain:**

A right lower lobe pneumonia
B acute diverticulitis
C Curtis–Fitz-Hugh syndrome
D Charcot's triad
E Beck's triad

33. **In otitis media**

A myringotomy is a recognized treatment
B amoxicillin is a reasonable antibiotic to use
C *Pneumococcus* is the commonest causative organism
D perforation of the tympanic membrane increases the pain
E epileptic fits may occur as a late complication

34. **Radiotherapy**

A is useful for pain relief in bone metastases
B increases the risk of fracture through a bone metastasis
C produces an acute relief of spinal cord compression due to its effects on bone
D causes nausea and vomiting in the majority of patients
E leads to sclerosis of lytic metastases within 6 weeks

35. **The following are signs of plasma volume overload:**

A bradycardia
B third heart sound
C reduced respiratory rate
D reduced jugular venous pressure
E hypotension

36. **Breast cancer**

A affects approximately 1 in 18 women in the UK
B is commoner in Ashkenazi Jews
C prognosis may be classified by the Edinburgh Prognostic Index
D decreases in incidence after the age of 75 years
E has a genetic aetiology in approximately 5–10% of patients

37. **Lignocaine**

A can be safely used with adrenaline when injecting the ear lobes
B is equally effective in inflamed areas, although more painful to inject
C at a dose of 2% gives twice as good analgesia as at 1%
D produces its analgesic affect faster with increased concentrations
E has a maximal dose of 10 mg/kg body weight

38. **Indications for a definitive airway include**

A the unconscious patient
B severe maxillofacial injuries
C a Glasgow Coma Score of 12
D stridor
E inhalation injuries

39. **In trauma to the pregnant patient**

A the initial treatment priorities remain the same as for a non-pregnant patient
B penetrating abdominal injuries are unlikely to directly affect the 10-week-old fetus
C amniotic fluid embolism may occur
D signs of hypovolaemia tend to occur earlier than in the non-pregnant patient
E unless a spinal injury is suspected, the patient should be transported on her right side

40. Which of the following statements are true concerning the detection and diagnosis of prostatic cancer?

A An elevation of prostate-specific antigen (PSA) is highly sensitive and specific for prostatic carcinoma.
B American blacks have an increased risk of prostatic carcinoma.
C Autopsy series would suggest that 10% of men in their 50s will have small latent prostatic cancers.
D Transrectal prostatic biopsy is indicated for a palpable 1 cm prostate nodule.
E Serum prostatic acid phosphatase remains the most useful tumour marker for prostatic carcinoma.

41. Recognized complications of renal transplantation include:

A renal artery stenosis
B renal failure
C hypertension
D hyperlipidaemia
E ureteric obstruction

42. The indications for thoracotomy in trauma include:

A haemothorax with initial drainage of 500 ml
B haemothorax with a bleeding rate of 200 ml/h for 4 consecutive hours
C cardiac tamponade
D tension pneumothorax
E empyema

43. The epiploic foramen (of Winslow)

A The anterior boundary is the free edge of the lesser omentum.
B The posterior boundary is the peritoneum over the duodenum.
C The inferior boundary is the transverse colon.
D The superior boundary is the caudate process of the liver.
E Is an important landmark in the treatment of liver haemorrhage.

44. Paget's disease

A of the breast is associated with underlying breast cancer in 50% of cases
B of the bone is associated with bone tumours
C of the bone affects 2–4% of the UK population in middle age
D of the bone is usually associated with both high serum calcium and high alkaline phosphatase
E of the breast may be diagnosed by a nipple scrape sent for cytology

45. **Cortisol**

A synthesis by the adrenals is controlled via cyclic AMP by ACTH
B reduces gluconeogenesis
C plasma level reaches a maximum at about midnight
D has considerable mineralocorticoid activity
E enhances production of angiotensinogen

46. **The following are true statements about bilirubin and its metabolites:**

A The daily production of bilirubin in a 70 kg adult is about 300 mg.
B Urobilins are colourless compounds.
C A fraction of urobilinogen is reabsorbed from the intestine and re-excreted through the liver.
D The conjugation of bilirubin is performed by enzymes called β-glucuronidases.
E Conjugated bilirubin is secreted into the bile by simple diffusion.

47. **The following statements concern potassium:**

A 30% of total body potassium is located in the extracellular compartment.
B Aldosterone increases active potassium secretion in the distal convoluted tubule.
C Hypokalaemia directly stimulates aldosterone secretion.
D Insulin causes potassium to enter the cell.
E Hypokalaemia will occur if the activity of the membrane-bound Na^+/K^+ pump is impaired.

48. **Hydrogen ion (H^+) homeostasis**

A Proteins are the principal buffer in urine.
B Hydrogen ions are secreted into the renal tubular lumen in exchange for potassium ions, so that they combine with the filtered bicarbonate.
C Bicarbonate is the most important buffer in the extracellular fluid.
D Ammonium ions (NH_4^+) can cross the membranes of renal tubular cells.
E The hydrogen ion concentration in arterial blood is directly proportional to the partial pressure of CO_2.

49. **The rectus abdominis muscle**

A crosses the costal margin
B usually has four tendinous intersections
C has a dual blood supply
D is used in breast reconstruction
E has a single nerve supply

50. Within the first week after severe trauma to a patient, there is an increase in

A aldosterone secretion
B urinary excretion of urea
C protein synthesis
D lipolysis
E antidiuretic hormone secretion

51. The palatine tonsil

A is separated from the superior constrictor muscle by lax connective tissue
B receives its blood supply from the facial artery
C lies anterior to the palatoglossal arch
D is separated from the glossopharyngeal nerve by the superior constrictor muscle of the pharynx
E receives blood supply from the ascending pharyngeal artery

52. Day-case surgery

A Most would regard the age of 85 years as the upper limit for day-surgery patients.
B Patients should preferably have a BMI < 30 for day surgery.
C Patients for day surgery should have an ASA score of I or II.
D Assessment of day patients is best performed by trained assessment nurses.
E Pilonidal sinus surgery and adult circumcisions are suitable day-case operations.

53. In the prophylaxis of deep venous thrombosis

A lower limb elevation is a simple useful method
B graduated compression stockings can safely be given to all patients undergoing surgery
C graduated compression stockings reduce the risk of DVT by 65–70%
D aspirin may be a useful pharmacological agent
E low-molecular-weight heparins are at least as efficacious as unfractionated heparin, with a small reduction in bleeding complications

54. *Helicobacter pylori*

A is present in 30% of the adult population
B is detected by the presence of labelled urea in the breath
C may be effectively eradicated with a combination of amoxicillin, clarithromycin and lansoprazole
D triple therapy is only effective in approximately 20% of infected patients
E is associated with gastric adenocarcinoma

55. **The following may be used to assess nutritional status:**

A height (metres) divided by weight (kg) squared (H/W^2)
B measurement of urinary urea over 24 hours
C bioelectrical impedence
D measurement of handgrip strength
E measurement of serum transferrin levels

56. **The following may be said of enteral feeding:**

A It is the route of choice if the gastrointestinal tract is intact and functioning.
B Elemental diets contain whole protein.
C Polymeric diets provide energy in the form of complex carbohydrates and fat.
D It is contraindicated in patients with intestinal obstruction.
E Feeding jejunostomies do not reduce the risk of pulmonary aspiration.

57. **The following are clinical manifestations of the multiple organ dysfunction syndrome (MODS):**

A hyperglycaemia
B fluid overload
C hypocapnia
D neuropathy
E gastrointestinal haemorrhage

58. **The following are recognized complications of laparoscopic surgery:**

A gas embolism
B bradycardia
C metabolic acidosis
D reduced cardiac output
E pneumatosis coli

59. **The following are well-recognized side-effects of cyclosporin:**

A tremors and convulsions
B hypotension
C gingival hypertrophy
D photosensitivity
E haemolytic anaemia

60. **The following statements regarding intravenous fluids and their components are true:**

A Dextrose saline is made up of 4% glucose and 0.9% sodium chloride.
B Hartmann's solution contains 131 mmol/l of sodium and 5 mmol/l of potassium.
C 3 litres of dextrose saline provide a similar amount of sodium as 1 litre of normal saline.
D Normal saline contains 155 mmol/l of chloride ions.
E 5% dextrose provides 200 kcal of energy.

61. **The following may affect delivery of oxygen to the tissues:**

A haemoglobin affinity for oxygen
B blood volume
C peripheral vascular resistance
D lung function
E type and duration of surgery

62. **The following are associated with a significantly prolonged thrombin time:**

A massive blood transfusion
B disseminated intravascular coagulation (DIC)
C vitamin K deficiency
D haemophilias
E idiopathic thrombocytopenic purpura

63. **The following are recognized adverse consequences of blood transfusion:**

A citrate toxicity
B Epstein–Barr virus transmission
C hepatitis C transmission
D prolonged bleeding
E hypersplenism

64. **Raynaud's phenomenon may be caused by the following:**

A cryoglobulinaemia
B scleroderma
C macroglobulinaemia
D thoracic outlet syndrome
E idiopathic thrombocytopenic purpura

65. **The long saphenous vein**

A is formed by the union of the dorsal vein of the great toe and the dorsal venous arch
B ascends posterior to the medial maleolus
C ascends posterior to the lateral maleolus
D lies deep to the crural fascia
E is now rarely used for coronary artery bypass graft surgery, as arterial grafts are better

66. **The following are associated with Crohn's disease:**

A vaginal ulcers
B erythema nodosum
C cirrhosis
D renal amyloidosis
E iritis

67. **The following relate to rectal prolapse:**

A It is unusual in infancy.
B Men are affected 20 times more commonly than women.
C It is more common after age 75 years.
D There is an association with mental impairment.
E It can be simulated by haemorrhoids and low rectal polyps.

68. **The following relate to the biliary system:**

A Courvoisier's law suggests that a palpable gallbladder is due to underlying cancer.
B Pringle's manoeuvre is used for biliary leaks.
C Charcot's triad consists of the following: palpable mass, pain and pyrexia.
D Gallstone ileus is the commonest reason for air in the biliary tree on plain abdominal X-rays.
E The majority of gallstones in the UK consist predominantly of cholesterol.

69. **During the approach to the submandibular gland, the following structures are found superficial to the gland:**

A hypoglossal nerve
B facial vein
C cervical branch of the facial nerve
D superior laryngeal nerve
E digastric muscle

70. The following nerves are at risk with the operations described:

A external branch of the superior laryngeal nerve – parathyroidectomy
B accessory nerve – lymph node biopsy from posterior triangle of the neck
C ilioinguinal nerve – low approach to femoral hernia repair
D sural nerve – varicose vein surgery
E intercostobrachial nerve – axillary lymph node clearance

71. Bladder cancer

A This most commonly presents with painless haematuria.
B Tumours of the urachal remnant are usually squamous cell carcinomas.
C Men are affected 10 times as often as women.
D If multiple small lesions are present, intravesical chemotherapy is a suitable treatment option.
E Stage T2 tumours do not penetrate the muscle wall of the bladder.

72. Muscles of the neck

A The strap muscles are supplied by the accessory nerve.
B The sternohyoid lies anterior to the sternothyroid.
C The omohyoid attaches to the scapular.
D The anterior belly of the digastric has a different nerve supply to the posterior belly.
E The mylohyoid is supplied by the facial nerve.

73. Head injuries

A Following the injury, nothing can be done to minimize the primary brain injury.
B Hyperventilation should be avoided during the initial management.
C A patient who withdraws normally, but cannot localize a painful stimulus, has a score of 5 on the Motor Response part of the Glasgow Coma Scale.
D Subdural haematomas are much more common than epidural haematomas.
E Ideally, a CT scan should be obtained in all significant head-injury patients if available.

74. The following concern postoperative pyrexia:

A Within 48 hours, pyrexia is commonly due to atelectasis.
B Within 3 days, it is unlikely to be due to an infective organism introduced during surgery.
C If >41 °C, it is most likely to be infectious.
D At 12 days, it is likely to be due to an anastomotic dehiscence.
E Pyrexia is is not associated with a postoperative deep venous thrombosis.

75. **The following concern pulmonary embolism:**

A The most common ECG abnormality is right-axis deviation.
B S1Q1T3 is a classical pattern highly suggestive of pulmonary embolism.
C It may present with atrial fibrillation.
D It classically presents 2 days after surgery.
E The most accurate investigation to confirm the diagnosis is a $\dot{V}/\dot{Q}$ scan.

76. **The following concern spinal cord injuries:**

A Brown–Séquard syndrome results from hemisection of the cord.
B Central cord syndrome is usually seen after a hyperflexion injury.
C Central cord syndrome is characterized by a greater loss of motor power in the lower limbs than in the upper limbs.
D Anterior cord syndrome is due to infarction of the cord in the territory of the anterior spinal artery.
E Anterior cord syndrome patients are typically paraplegic.

77. **Indications for cardiopulmonary bypass include**

A supradiaphragmatic aortic surgery
B hypothermia
C chronic cardiac failure
D pneumonectomy
E coronary artery bypass grafting

78. **Combination chemotherapy**

A Combination chemotherapy can potentially cure multiple metastases, whereas radiotherapy and surgery cannot.
B Neoadjuvant chemotherapy refers to the latest combination of cytotoxics being given following surgery.
C Combination chemotherapy can potentially cure Hodgkin's disease and germ cell tumours.
D It has a poor outcome with melanoma and soft tissue sarcomas.
E It should ideally contain drugs that have similar mechanisms of action.

79. Lower-limb amputation

A If transfemoral (above-knee), amputation results in 50% of patients being able to walk again.
B Ideal stumps should be conical in shape and heal by primary intention.
C Scars should transmit pressure during ambulation.
D The PAM (pneumatic postamputation mobility) aid should be applied to the stump approximately 4 weeks after surgery if the wound has healed.
E Lower-limb amputation is performed in approximately 10% of diabetic patients during their lifetime.

80. Splenectomy

A This is indicated for autoimmune thrombocytopenia.
B It is indicated for capsular tears that are 2 cm deep into the parenchyma.
C Patients should be vaccinated against *Meningococcus*.
D Patients are at a higher risk of infection from encapsulated organisms postoperatively.
E Postoperative oral penicillin prophylaxis is of proven value in children.

81. Peripheral nerve injury

A A crushing injury is most likely to be neurotmesis.
B The axon grows at 1 mm/week after nerve section.
C The proximal axon undergoes Wallerian degeneration.
D Transient impairment of conduction is known as neuropraxia.
E Primary nerve repair is still preferable after inadvertent division of a nerve during a contaminated operation.

82. In the healing of fractures

A the cells of the deeper layer of the periosteum have osteogenic potential
B the pH of the uniting fracture starts to decrease after about 10 days
C the bone ends show osteoporosis in the early stages of fracture healing
D healing is impaired in hyperparathyroidism
E globules of fat may enter the disrupted vascular spaces and embolize

83. **Cholinergic impulses in the autonomic nervous system produce**

A increased intestinal motility
B gallbladder relaxation
C detrusor muscle relaxation
D penile erection
E a decrease in atrial contractility

84. **The brain**

A The brain receives 5% of the cardiac output.
B It compensates for a rise in intracranial pressure by losing CSF in the lumbar thecal sac.
C It receives approximately 750 ml blood flow per minute.
D The intracranial pressure is normally 0–10 mmHg.
E The intracranial pressure is directly proportional to the volume of skull contents.

85. **The clinical signs of cervical cord injury include**

A priapism and decreased anal sphincter tone
B Cullen sign
C tachycardia (if not hypovolaemic)
D urinary retention
E hypertension

86. **Recognized consequences of endotoxic shock include**

A adult respiratory distress syndrome (ARDS)
B warm peripheries
C hypothermia
D interstitial oedema
E gastrointestinal haemorrhage

87. **Anterior shoulder dislocation**

A is less common than posterior dislocation
B can be treated using Kocher's manoeuvre
C is a recognized cause of axillary nerve palsy
D is usually subcoracoid
E usually presents with the arm in the adduction position

88. The following relate to the cell cycle:

A Cells are most sensitive to ionizing radiation during S phase.
B DNA synthesis is confined to S phase.
C During G_1 phase, the cells are metabolically inactive.
D The total duration of the cell cycle in normal tissues is constant.
E The cells of solid tumours in humans all proceed through the cell cycle in the same phase.

89. *Staphylococcus aureus* is usually responsible for abscess formation in the following sites:

A appendix
B axilla
C finger pulp
D ischiorectal area
E breast

90. Cell-mediated (type IV) hypersensitivity reactions

A $CD8^+$ cells recognize antigen in conjunction with MHC class II molecules.
B The reaction is seen in the rejection of a transplanted kidney.
C The reaction takes 4–10 hours to develop.
D Sensitized $CD4^+$ cells produce lymphokines that help macrophages to kill intracellular parasites.
E Cell-mediated immunity has been implicated in the protection against some cancers.

Practice Paper 3

Clinical Problem Solving – EMQs

- This paper consists of 150 extended matching items.
- Questions consist of a theme, a list of options, an instruction and a variable number of clinical situations.
- For each of the clinical situations, you should choose the **single most likely option** according to the instruction.
- It is possible for one option to be the answer to more than one of the clinical situations.
- Marks will not be deducted for a wrong answer. Equally, you will not gain a mark if you mark more than one option.
- Only answers that are clearly struck horizontally across the correct response will guarantee a mark.
- Faint marking may be misread. All scores within 5 marks of the pass mark will be scrutinized.

Practice Paper 3: Part 2 – EMQs in Clinical Problem Solving

Theme: Blood transfusion

Options

A Group A Rh D-negative
B Group A Rh D-positive
C Group B Rh D-positive
D Group O Rh D-negative
E Anti-D immunoglobulin
F Iron sulphate tablets

For each of the patients described below, select the single most appropriate product from the list above. Each option may be used once, more than once or not at all.

1. A 60-year-old man with blood group A Rh D-negative and Hb of 6.0.
2. A 20-year-old woman with blood group B Rh D-negative and Hb of 6.0.
3. A mother with blood group A Rh D-negative and Hb of 10.1 having just given birth to a baby with blood group A Rh D-positive.
4. A postoperative patient with blood group A Rh D-negative and Hb of 9.2.
5. A 50-year-old man with blood group O Rh D-positive and Hb of 6.0.

Theme: Breast disease

Options
A Fibroadenoma
B Fat necrosis
C Fibrocystic disease
D Duct papilloma
E Ductal carcinoma in situ
F Invasive breast cancer
G Duct ectasia
H Paget's disease

For each of the patients described below, select the single most appropriate diagnosis above. Each option may be used once, more than once or not at all.

6. A 20-year-old woman with a 3 cm discrete, mobile, firm mass in the upper inner quadrant of the left breast.
7. A 45-year-old woman with a 3-month history of right-sided bloody nipple discharge and new inversion of the nipple.
8. A 70-year-old woman with a hard, irregular 3 cm lump in the left breast with overlying skin dimpling. Core biopsy showed plasma cells and fibrosis, B2.
9. A 50-year-old woman who smokes 20 cigarettes/day presents with a year-long history of left breast pain and green nipple discharge.
10. A 65-year-old woman with a 3 cm firm lump in the right breast and another 2 cm lump in the right axilla. FNA of both lumps revealed C5.

Theme: Groin lumps

Options
A Testicular cancer
B Varicocoele
C Direct inguinal hernia
D Indirect inguinal hernia
E Hydrocoele
F Hydrocoele of the cord
G Epididymal cyst
H Epididymo-orchitis
I Testicular torsion

For each of the patients described below, select the single most appropriate diagnosis above. Each option may be used once, more than once or not at all.

11. A 25-year-old man with a soft swelling in the left scrotum, only palpable on standing, feels like a bag of worms.
12. A 25-year-old man with a 2-day history of gradual onset pain in the right testicle. On examination the testicle is red, swollen and tender to touch.

13. A 25-year-old man with soft swelling in the right scrotum. On examination it has a positive cough impulse and the examiner is unable to get above the lump.
14. A 25-year-old man with a diffusely enlarged right scrotum, soft and non-tender to examine that brightly transilluminates.
15. A 25-year-old man with a painless, enlarging lump in the left scrotum. On examination there is a 2 cm firm nodule but also extensive swelling of the scrotum that brightly transilluminates.

Theme: Neck lumps

Options

A Multinodular goitre
B Salivary gland calculus
C Lymph node
D Epidermal cyst – Sebaceous cyst
E Pleomorphic adenoma
F Branchial cyst
G Cystic hygroma
H Dermoid cyst
I Thyroglossal cyst

For each of the patients described below, select the single most appropriate diagnosis above. Each option may be used once, more than once or not at all.

16. A 12-year-old boy with a 3 cm soft, fluctuant swelling on the left side below the angle of the mandible that brightly transilluminates.
17. A 30-year-old woman with a 2 cm firm lump just to the left of the midline in the lower neck that moves on swallowing but does not move on protruding the tongue.
18. A 40-year-old man has an intermittent uncomfortable swelling on the left side of his neck below the angle of the mandible – usually during meal times.
19. A 20-year-old woman with a 1 cm lump in the midline of her neck that rises on protruding the tongue.
20. A 30-year-old man with a 2 cm firm nodule beneath the angle of the mandible that is fixed to the skin and has a small punctum.

Theme: Thyroid disease

Options
A Graves' disease
B Hashimoto's disease
C Multinodular goitre
D Thyroid cancer
E Functional follicular adenoma
F de Quervain's thyroiditis
G Endemic goitre
H Riedel's thyroiditis

For each of the patients described below, select the single most appropriate diagnosis above. Each option may be used once, more than once or not at all.

21. A 36-year-old woman with recent weight loss notices a discrete nodule on the left side of the midline of her neck. Her serum TSH is unmeasurable.
22. A 50-year-old woman with a long history of a swelling in the midline of her lower neck sees her GP as she is having increasing difficulty swallowing. TFTs are normal.
23. A 29-year-old woman complains of diarrhoea, weight loss and sweatiness. Her TSH is low, the T_4 level is elevated and thyroid-stimulating antibodies are positive.
24. A 40-year-old woman presents with a mildly tender generalized swelling of the thyroid gland. She has put on weight recently despite being on a diet. She also complains of constipation. Her TSH is raised and she also has a macrocytic anaemia.
25. A 60-year-old man presents to the local clinic with a massive thyroid swelling. He is a farmer in the foothills of the Himalayas of Nepal. The swelling has been increasing for many years, but now his grandchildren have started teasing him about it. His TSH is mildly raised and the T_4 is at the low end of normal.

Theme: Thyroid cancer

Options
A Anaplastic
B Follicular
C Medullary
D Papillary
E Lymphoma

For each of the patients described below, select the single most appropriate diagnosis above. Each option may be used once, more than once or not at all.

26. A 65-year-old woman who previously underwent cervical exploration for hyperparathyroidism notices a painless lump in the thyroid with associated lymphadenopathy.

27. A 45-year-old radiographer with a slowly growing lump in the thyroid and cervical lymphadenopathy.
28. An 85-year-old woman with a rapidly growing lump in the neck, new-onset hoarseness of the voice and a pathological fracture of the femoral neck.
29. A 10-year-old girl with a small lump in the thyroid. FNA shows malignant cells.
30. A 60-year-old woman taking thyroxine for long-standing Hashimoto's thyroiditis notices an increasing size of the goiter and unilateral cervical lymphadenopathy.

Theme: Hepatobiliary disease

Options

A Plain X-ray
B Ultrasound scan
C Contrast CT
D Endoscopic retrograde cholangiopancreatogram (ERCP)
E MRI (MRCP)
F Percutaneous transhepatic cholangiogram (PTC)

For each of the clinical scenarios described below, select the single most appropriate investigation that should be performed next from the list above. Each option may be used once, more than once or not at all.

31. A 40-year-old woman with a 2-day history of right upper quadrant pain, fevers and vomiting. Her liver function tests (LFTs) and amylase are normal.
32. A 30-year-old alcoholic man admitted 3 days prior with epigastric pain and vomiting. Amylase on admission was 1500. He now has spiking temperatures and his white cell count is rising. His LFTs are becoming more deranged.
33. A 70-year-old woman with a long history of gallstones presents to A&E with colicky abdominal pain and vomiting. Her abdomen is distended and bowel sounds are high-pitched.
34. A 55-year-old man with right upper quadrant pain and vomiting. Bilirubin = 120, alkaline phosphatase = 300, ALT = 90. Ultrasound showed dilated hepatic ducts and CBD = 2 cm; a 1 cm stone was seen in the distal CBD.
35. A 60-year-old woman with a 6-month history of upper abdominal discomfort and weight loss. CA 19-9 markedly raised. She presents with deep jaundice, and an ultrasound shows dilated hepatic ducts. ERCP was unsuccessful at passing a tight CBD narrowing.

Theme: Hip fractures

Options
A Dynamic hip screw
B Total hip replacement
C Cemented hemiarthroplasty
D Uncemented hemiarthroplasty
E Cannulated screws
F Traction
G Intramedullary hip screw
H External fixator

For each of the clinical scenarios described below, select the single most appropriate procedure that should be performed from the list above. Each option may be used once, more than once or not at all.

36. A 75-year-old woman trips at home and presents with an extracapsular fracture of the neck of the left femur.
37. A 30-year-old man is a passenger in a car involved in an RTA. He is hit from the side. Pelvic X-ray shows an intracapsular fracture of the neck of the left femur.
38. A 60-year-old woman with severe rheumatoid arthritis affecting both hips and knees falls whilst shopping and presents to A&E with a shortened, externally rotated left leg. X-ray shows an intracapsular fracture of the neck of the femur.
39. A 90-year-old man with severe COPD falls when walking back from the bathroom. X-ray reveals an extracapsular fracture of the neck of the femur.
40. A 65-year-old man is a pedestrian hit by a car. He has an extracapsular fracture of the neck of the femur extending into a spiral fracture of the proximal shaft of the femur.

Theme: Flexor tendon injuries

Options
A Zone 1
B Zone 2
C Zone 3
D Zone 4
E Zone 5

For each of the scenarios described below, select the single most appropriate zone of injury from the list above. Each option may be used once, more than once or not at all.

41. A laceration across the volar side of the metacarpal–phalyngeal joint with division of the FDS tendon.

42. A laceration across the volar aspect of the distal interphalyngeal joint with division of the FDP tendon.
43. A laceration proximal to the flexor retinaculum with division of several flexor tendons.
44. Division of the FDP tendon between the A1 and A2 pulleys.
45. Division of the FDS to ring finger within the carpal tunnel.

Theme: Salter–Harris classification of fractures

Options

A Type 1
B Type 2
C Type 3
D Type 4
E Type 5

For each of the scenarios described below, select the single most appropriate type of fracture from the list above. Each option may be used once, more than once or not at all.

46. An oblique fracture extending through the metaphysis, epiphyseal plate and epiphysis into the joint.
47. A crush injury to the epiphyseal plate that is often missed on initial X-ray.
48. A fracture through the epiphyseal plate that includes a small flake of the metaphysis.
49. A fracture straight through the epiphyseal plate with separation of the epiphysis from the metaphysis.
50. A fracture through the epiphyseal plate and epiphysis and extending into the joint.
51. The most common type of growth plate fracture.

Theme: Lower limb injuries

Options
A L5 root
B L4 root
C S1 root
D Sciatic nerve
E Common peroneal nerve
F Deep peroneal nerve
G Superficial peroneal nerve
H Tibial nerve
I Femoral nerve
J Sural nerve
K Saphenous nerve
L Superior gluteal nerve
M Obturator nerve

For each of the scenarios below, choose the most appropriate level of injury from the list above. Each option may be used once, more than once or not at all.

52. A patient with numbness on the sole of her foot and inability to plantarflex the foot following total knee replacement.
53. A patient with acute back pain, numbness in the first web space of the left foot and inability to lift up the left big toe.
54. A patient with a fractured fibula who cannot dorsiflex the same foot and has numbness in the first web space.
55. A patient with numbness on the lateral side of his lower leg following total hip replacement.
56. A patient with numbness on the lateral side of the foot following varicose vein surgery.

Theme: Upper limb injuries

Options
A Musculocutaneous nerve
B Median nerve
C Accessory nerve
D Radial nerve
E Ulnar nerve
F Anterior interosseous nerve
G Axillary nerve
H C5/C6 nerve roots
I Posterior cord of the brachial plexus
J C7/C8 nerve roots

For each of the scenarios below, choose the most appropriate level of injury from the list above. Each option may be used once, more than once or not at all.

57. A 70-year-old man with a fracture of the humerus is unable to extend his wrist.

58. A 25-year-old man falls from his motorbike onto his right shoulder and now holds his right arm in a characteristic 'waiter's tip' position.
59. A 7-year-old boy falls from a climbing frame and has a painful swollen elbow. His thumb feel like 'pins and needles'.
60. A patient has had a plate put on his proximal radius. When asked to perform the 'OK' sign with this hand, he cannot make a circle but pushes the pulps of the index finger and thumb together. On closer examination, he cannot flex the distal interphalyngeal joint of his index finger or the interphalyngeal joint of his thumb.
61. A patient with a dislocated shoulder has a patch of numbness over the lower part of the corresponding deltoid muscle.

Theme: Blood gases

Options

A Metabolic acidosis (uncompensated)
B Metabolic alkalosis (uncompensated)
C Respiratory acidosis (uncompensated)
D Respiratory alkalosis (uncompensated)
E Metabolic acidosis (compensated)
F Metabolic alkalosis (compensated)
G Respiratory acidosis (compensated)
H Respiratory alkalosis (compensated)

For each of the blood gas results below, choose the most appropriate derangement from the list above. Each option may be used once, more than once or not at all.

62. pH = 7.99, pO_2 = 9 kPa, pCO_2 = 2.8 kPa, BE = 1.0.
63. pH = 6.91, pO_2 = 11 kPa, pCO_2 = 2.8 kPa, BE = −9.5.
64. pH = 7.49, pO_2 = 10 kPa, pCO_2 = 3.0, BE = +4.5.

Theme: Rectal bleeding in children

Options
A Haemorrhoids
B Necrotizing enterocolitis
C Intussusception
D Meckel's diverticulum
E Inflammatory bowel disease
F Anal fissure
G Gastroenteritis
H Vascular malformation
I Bowel polyps

For each of the clinical scenarios below, select the single most appropriate diagnosis from the list above. Each option may be used once, more than once or not at all.

65. A 5-year-old girl who cries after opening her bowels (infrequently). Her mother has noticed bright red blood on the paper.
66. A 2-week-old baby (born at 28 weeks) is noticed to have a distended abdomen, vomiting and rectal bleeding whilst on the neonatal unit.
67. A 10-year-old boy noticed that he has been passing red blood mixed in with his stool. He has no pain and is otherwise well. A technetium-99 m scan shows increased uptake in the suprapubic region.
68. A 14-year-old girl complains of a 6-month history of diarrhoea with occasional episodes of rectal bleeding. She has lost over 1 stone in weight. Of note, she returned from a 2-week holiday to India 1 month ago.
69. A 9-month-old boy is brought to A&E. His mother says that he has been crying, vomiting and intermittently drawing up his legs for the past 6 hours. There is blood mixed with mucus in his nappy.

Theme: ATLS classification of haemorrhage

Options
A Class I
B Class II
C Class III
D Class IV

For each of the scenarios below, select the single most appropriate answer from the list above. Each option may be used once, more than once or not at all.

70. A 20-year-old motorcyclist is brought in to A&E following an RTA. He has an open femoral fracture. Pulse 120/min, BP 110/90, respiratory rate 25/min, urine output 30 ml/h.

71. A 70 kg man has bled approximately 2 litres into his peritoneal cavity following traumatic rupture of his spleen.
72. A 15-year-old girl has a nose bleed following an RTA. Estimated blood loss is 5% of her circulating volume.
73. A 50-year-old man with multiple injuries following an RTA. No witnesses available. He is cold and drowsy. His pulse is 170/min, BP 60/45.
74. A 30-year-old woman bleeds heavily post-partum. She is tachycardic, but her systolic blood pressure is no different from that previously measured.

Theme: Burns

Options
A 1%
B 9%
C 18%
D 27%
E 36%
F 45%
G 54%

From the list above, estimate the percentage of total surface area involved for each of the burns below. Each option may be used once, more than once or not at all.

75. A man with full-thickness burns circumferentially to the whole of his right arm.
76. A man with full-thickness burns circumferentially to the whole of his right leg.
77. A man with full-thickness burns to the whole posterior aspect of his leg.
78. A man with full-thickness burns to his head and face.
79. A man with full-thickness burns to the whole of his perineum.

Theme: Urological symptoms

Options
A Infective urethritis
B Bladder calculi
C Prostatic adenocarcinoma
D Posterior urethral valve
E Urethral stricture
F Benign prostatic hyperplasia
G Urinary tract infection
H Ureteric calculi

For each of the clinical scenarios below, select the single most appropriate diagnosis from the list above. Each option may be used once, more than once or not at all.

80. A 55-year-old man who complains of worsening nocturia associated with terminal dribbling and hesitancy. PSA is 4.5 ng/ml.
81. A 25-year-old man who complains of a poor urinary stream. He was treated for an NSU 6 months previously.
82. An 80-year-old man with a long-term catheter who presents with haematuria, vomiting and suprapubic discomfort.
83. A 30-year-old man who presents with haematuria, vomiting and pain in his left side and testicle.
84. A 50-year-old man who presents with acute urinary retention. Urine analysis shows blood ++, leucocytes ++. A urinary catheter is passed (residual is 800 ml). 30 minutes later the catheter falls out. A second catheter again falls out 1 hour later.

Theme: Peripheral vascular disease

Options
A Femoral–popliteal bypass
B Above-knee amputation
C Below-knee amputation
D Lumbar sympathectomy
E Balloon angioplasty with or without stent
F Femoral embolectomy
G Femoral–femoral crossover
H Femoral–distal bypass
I Axillo–bifemoral bypass
J Aorto–bifemoral bypass
K Aorto–biiliac bypass

For each of the clinical scenarios below, choose the single most appropriate treatment from the list above. Each option may be used once, more than once or not at all.

85. A 40-year-old man who complains of bilateral buttock claudication and impotence. Angiogram shows a stenosis of the distal aorta.

86. A 70-year-old man with severe COPD who complains of rest pain in both legs. Angiogram shows extensive, severe bilateral stenosis of the distal external iliac arteries.
87. A 70-year-old man presents with two large ischaemic, infected ulcers on his left foot. A plain X-ray shows lucency of the bone underlying the ulcers. Angiogram shows moderate stenosis of the superficial femoral artery, severe stenosis of the popliteal artery and moderate to severe stenosis of all three vessels below the knee.
88. A 60-year-old man who is a smoker and has hypertension and atrial fibrillation presents to A&E with an acutely painful, white leg. Only his femoral pulse is palpable on that side.
89. A 59-year-old woman presents with a 1-year history of worsening claudication in her left leg. She is now unable to walk more than 20 yards. Angiogram shows a 3 cm severe stenosis midway along the superficial femoral artery.
90. A 65-year-old man presents with rest pain in his right foot. He has no pulses palpable below the femoral. Angiogram shows extensive disease all through his superficial femoral and popliteal artery but with collateral filling of a good-calibre anterior tibial vessel.

Theme: Prostate cancer

Options

A Radical prostatectomy
B External-beam radiotherapy
C Brachytherapy
D TURP
E Hormonal therapy
F Watch and wait

For each of the clinical scenarios below, choose the single most appropriate treatment from the options listed above. Each option may be used once, more than once or not at all.

91. A 70-year-old man is found to have a raised PSA. Biopsies from a TURP show a well-differentiated adenocarcinoma, and further investigations show no evidence of metastatic disease.
92. A 50-year-old man complains of urinary hesitancy, terminal dribbling and poor flow. Digital rectal examination reveals a hard, craggy prostate. Biopsies reveal extensive, poorly differentiated adenocarcinoma. There is no evidence of extraprostatic spread of disease.
93. A 70-year-old man presents with urinary incontinence. He is found to have locally advanced prostate cancer with pelvic and spinal metastases.
94. A 60-year-old man with stage D prostate cancer. When he comes for his regular goserelin (Zoladex) injections, he complains of lower back pain. A plain X-ray shows sclerotic lesions in the L4 and L5 vertebrae.

Theme: Jaundice

Options

A Prehepatic jaundice
B Hepatocellular disease
C Gallstone in the common bile duct
D Biliary colic
E Mirizzi syndrome
F Carcinoma of the head of the pancreas
G Cholangiocarcinoma
H Sclerosing cholangitis
I Pancreatitis
J Gallstone ileus

For each of the clinical scenarios below, choose the single most likely diagnosis from the list above. Each option may be used once, more than once or not at all.

95. A 60-year-old woman presents to her GP with vague abdominal pain. She is found to be jaundiced, and on examination she has a palpable enlarged gallbladder.
96. A 35-year-old woman presents to A&E with right upper quadrant pain and jaundice associated with vomiting. Bilirubin is 200 μmol/l, ALT 150 u/l, alkaline phosphatase 1030 u/l and amylase 150 u/l. Ultrasound of the abdomen showed dilated intrahepatic ducts and a scarred, shrunken gallbladder, but the CBD was not visualized due to body habitus.
97. A 26-year-old man returns from a holiday in Thailand. He presents to A&E with a fever and is noticed to be jaundiced. His bilirubin is 75 μmol/l (unconjugated). The rest of his LFTs are normal.
98. A 35-year-old woman presents to A&E with right upper quadrant pain, vomiting and fever. She is jaundiced. Bilirubin is 150 μmol/l, ALT 160 u/l, alkaline phosphatase 650 u/l, WBC 19 and amylase 110 u/l. An ultrasound shows a thick-walled gallbladder containing lots of stones and pericystic fluid. The intrahepatic ducts are dilated and the CBD has a diameter of 8 mm.
99. A 40-year-old man has his LFTs measured: bilirubin 120 μmol/l, ALT 3100 u/l, alkaline phosphatase 160 u/l, γ-GT 150 u/l.
100. A 45-year-old woman has ulcerative colitis. She attends the clinic and says her eyes are looking yellow. On examination, there is tenderness in the right upper quadrant but no masses. Bilirubin is 190 μmol/l, ALT 60 u/l, alkaline phosphatase 2040 u/l and γ-GT 500 u/l.

Theme: The paediatric abdomen

Options

A Meckel's diverticulum
B Meconium ileus
C Intussusception
D Hirschsprung's disease
E Pyloric stenosis
F Gastro-oesophageal reflux disease
G Malrotation volvulus
H Duodenal atresia

For each of the clinical scenarios below, choose the single most likely diagnosis from the list above. Each option may be used once, more than once or not at all.

101. A 3-year-old boy presents with dark red rectal bleeding and anaemia but is otherwise well. Examination is entirely normal.
102. A 6-week-old boy is brought to A&E with milky projectile vomiting and is found to have a metabolic alkalosis.
103. A 5-day-old baby girl with Down syndrome is brought to A&E severely dehydrated with persistant vomiting. Plain abdominal X-ray shows a double bubble.
104. A 6-week-old girl presents with intermittent bilious vomiting and colic. She has a tender abdomen but no masses.
105. A 9-month-old boy presents with bilious vomiting, colic and rectal bleeding. There is a sausage-shaped mass on the right side of the abdomen.

Theme: Abdominal pain

Options

A Pancreatitis
B Pyelonephritis
C Ureteric calculus
D Reflux oesophagitis
E Cholecystitis
F Adult polycystic kidney disease
G Hypernephroma
H Abdominal aortic aneurysm
I Urinary tract infection
J Appendicitis
K Perforated duodenal ulcer

For each of the clinical scenarios below, choose the single most likely diagnosis from the list above. Each option may be used once, more than once or not at all.

106. A 25-year-old woman presents to A&E with left loin pain and a fever. Her urine dipstick shows blood, leucocytes and nitrites.
107. A 50-year-old man complains of left loin pain for the past 2 weeks. Urine dipstick shows blood++. He has a palpable mass in the left loin.
108. A 65-year-old man presents to A&E after collapsing in the street with severe left loin pain. On examination, he has a pulse of 120/min and a BP of 90/40. His amylase is 400 iu/l.
109. A 65-year-old woman with rheumatoid arthritis presents to A&E with severe abdominal pain and dark brown vomiting. She has marked tenderness and guarding, especially in the upper abdomen. WBC 24, amylase 300 iu/l.
110. A 16-year-old girl is brought to her GP with a 2-day history of vague suprapubic/pelvic discomfort, anorexia and vomiting. She is tender in the right iliac fossa but has no guarding. Urinalysis shows leucocytes.

Theme: Gastrointestinal investigations

Options

A Proctoscopy
B Ultrasound scan
C Oesophagogastroduodenoscopy
D Colonoscopy
E Mesenteric angiogram
F Laparoscopy
G Laparotomy
H Labelled red cell scan
I CT scan
J Barium enema
K MRI scan

For each of the clinical scenarios below, choose the single most appropriate investigation from the list above. Each option may be used once, more than once or not at all.

111. A 40-year-old man complains of a burning epigastric pain and nausea. He is a smoker and a heavy drinker.
112. A 50-year-old man presents to A&E with a very large PR bleed (passing clots of red blood). He is profoundly shocked, pulse 160/min, BP 90/50.
113. A 40-year-old obese woman complains of 'indigestion'-like pain in the epigatrium and right upper quadrant after eating, associated with nausea.
114. A 30-year-old man has noticed blood dripping into the pan after opening his bowels. There are also streaks of fresh blood on the paper. Apart from constipation, he is otherwise well.
115. A 65-year-old woman presents to A&E with profuse bright red haematemesis. She is tachycardic at 190/min with a BP of 95/40. Her past medical history is that she had an open cholecystectomy 10 years ago and a laparotomy for small-bowel obstruction 5 years ago. The gastroenterology registrar has attempted an OGD, but is unsuccessful due to the volume of blood.
116. A 20-year-old woman is seen in the outpatient clinic with bright red rectal bleeding. Rigid sigmoidoscopy is normal.

Theme: Upper gastrointestinal surgery

Options

A Billroth I partial gastrectomy
B Billroth II Polya gastrectomy
C Total radical gastrectomy
D Distal pancreatectomy
E Proximal pancreatectomy
F Total pancreatectomy
G Hepatectomy
H Cholecystectomy
I Whipple's procedure
J Duodenectomy
K Gastroduodenal bypass
L A triple-bypass procedure
M Vagotomy and pyloroplasty

For each of the clinical scenarios below, choose the single most appropriate operation from the list above. Each option may be used once, more than once or not at all.

117. A 50-year-old woman with a 3 cm periampullary cholangiocarcinoma but no local or distant spread.
118. An 80-year-old man presents with dehydration, profuse non-bile-stained vomiting and a metabolic alkalosis. A CT scan shows a large tumour of the pylorus with spread to the surrounding lymph nodes and a metastasis in the liver.
119. A 50-year-old man complained of dyspepsia despite prolonged proton-pump inhibitor use and *H. pylori* eradication. At OGD, he is found to have an ulcer with raised edges high on the lesser curve of the stomach. Biopsies show signet-ring cells.
120. A 60-year-old man complained of dyspepsia despite prolonged proton-pump inhibitor use and *H. pylori* eradication. At OGD, he is found to have a deep punched-out ulcer in the first part of the duodenum. Biopsies show granulation tissue.
121. A 55-year-old man presents to A&E with obstructive jaundice. A CT scan shows a mass within the head of the pancreas but no spread into the portal vein or to the local lymph nodes.
122. A 55-year-old man presents to A&E with obstructive jaundice. A CT scan shows a mass within the head of the pancreas but with extensive spread into the portal vein (causing thrombosis) and involving the local lymph nodes.

Theme: Colorectal surgery

Options

A Small-bowel resection
B Right hemicolectomy
C Extended right hemicolectomy
D Transverse colectomy
E Left hemicolectomy
F Extended left hemicolectomy
G Sigmoid colectomy and primary anastomosis
H Hartmann's procedure
I Subtotal colectomy
J Panproctocolectomy
K Anterior resection
L Abdominoperineal resection
M Palliative defunctioning colostomy
N Watch and wait

For each of the clinical scenarios below, choose the single most appropriate option from the list above. Each option may be used once, more than once or not at all.

123. A 65-year-old woman is investigated for anaemia and weight loss. She is found to have a tumour in the caecum with no evidence of distal spread.
124. A 70-year-old woman is admitted with abdominal pain, distension and vomiting. Her symptoms do not settle with conservative treatment, so a laparotomy is performed. At surgery, a large tumour is felt in the sigmoid colon with gross dilatation of the descending colon. There is no evidence of any metastases.
125. A 60-year-old man complains of a constant desire to pass stool and has noticed several episodes of bleeding per rectum. On digital examination, he has a craggy mass at the anorectal junction. A CT scan shows no metastatic disease.
126. A 60-year-old man is investigated for bleeding per rectum. At colonoscopy, a suspicious polypoid mass is found at the splenic flexure. Biopsies taken confirm adenocarcinoma. A CT shows bulky nodes in the mesentery nearby, but the liver is clear.
127. A 20-year-old man attends the outpatient clinic. His father, uncle and sister have all died of colorectal cancer. He has no symptoms of bowel disease, but when a colonoscopy was performed he had hundreds of tubular polyps throughout the bowel. Biopsy of several of these lesions showed them to be benign adenomatous polyps.

Theme: Skin disease

Options
A Benign mole
B Malignant melanoma
C Basal cell carcinoma
D Epidermal cyst
E Squamous cell carcinoma
F Seborrhoeic keratosis
G Squamous cell papilloma
H Histiocytoma
I Marjolin's ulcer
J Keratoacanthoma

For each of the scenarios below, choose the single most appropriate option from the list above. Each option may be used once, more than once or not at all.

128. A 70-year-old woman goes to the GP because she has noticed that a raised pigmented lesion on her back has started bleeding. On examination, there are several raised brown nodules with variable pigmentation and a waxy appearance. One of them is partly lifted and is bleeding at the base.
129. A 70-year-old woman is seen at the clinic. She has a 1 cm diameter lesion on the left side of her nose that has been growing for the past 6 months. It has a pearly appearance with some telangectasia.
130. An 80-year-old woman has a 4 cm diameter lesion on her right shin. It has been steadily growing for the last year. It has a central area of crusting, under which is a deep ulcer. Around the periphery is a rolled, indurated margin.
131. A 30-year-old man sees the GP because a 2 cm nodule on his back has been increasing in size and bleeds when traumatized. It is darkly pigmented and is asymmetric.
132. A 40-year-old woman presents to the minor operations clinic. She has a 2 cm diameter firm brown nodule on her leg that occasionally itches. She thinks it started as a mosquito bite.

Theme: Diarrhoea

Options

A Crohn's disease
B Ulcerative colitis
C Viral gastroenteritis
D Appendicitis
E Amoebic dysentery
F Diverticulitis
G Coeliac disease
H Chronic pancreatitis
I Blind-loop syndrome
J Carcinoma of the head of the pancreas
K Typhoid fever
L Carcinoma of the colon

For each of the clinical scenarios below, choose the single most likely diagnosis from the list above. Each option may be used once, more than once or not at all.

133. A 20-year-old man is admitted to A&E with a 2-day history of abdominal pain, anorexia and diarrhoea. He has vomited twice and has a temperature of 38°C. He is tender in the lower abdomen and on per rectum examination.
134. A 60-year-old woman complains to her GP of weight loss, jaundice, dark urine and frequent loose stools that do not flush.
135. A 55-year-old woman is seen in the outpatient clinic as a followup after a Polya-type gastrectomy for gastric cancer. She complains of persistent diarrhoea for the past 6 months, but no vomiting. She is found to have a macrocytic anaemia.
136. A 60-year-old man returns from a holiday to India. He has a high temperature and bloody diarrhoea. On sigmoidoscopy, he has severely inflamed rectal mucosa.
137. A 40-year-old alcoholic man complains of epigastric and back pain associated with persistent pale loose stools. He has lost weight and appears anaemic.

Theme: Carcinogens

Options

A Soot
B Asbestos
C β-Naphthylamine
D UV light
E Arsenic
F Aflatoxin
G Ionizing radiation
H Nickel
I Benzopyrene
J Vinyl chloride monomer

For each of the tumours below, choose the single most implicated carcinogen from the list above. Each option may be used once, more than once or not at all.

138. Hepatocellular carcinoma.
139. Bladder cancer.
140. Malignant melanoma.
141. Thyroid cancer.
142. Mesothelioma.
143. Squamous cell carcinoma of the scrotum.

Theme: Viral carcinogens

Options

A Hepatitis A virus
B Hepatitis B virus
C Hepatitis C virus
D Epstein–Barr virus
E Human papillomavirus
F Herpes simplex virus
G HTLV-I
H Human immunodeficiency virus
I Cytomegalovirus

For each of the tumours below, choose the single most implicated virus from the list above. Each option may be used once, more than once or not at all.

144. Kaposi sarcoma.
145. Hepatocellular carcinoma.
146. Burkitt lymphoma.
147. Leukaemia.
148. Cervical carcinoma.
149. Nasopharyngeal carcinoma.
150. Hodgkin lymphoma.

Practice Paper 4

Clinical Problem Solving – EMQs

- This paper consists of 150 extended matching items.
- Questions consist of a theme, a list of options, an instruction and a variable number of clinical situations.
- For each of the clinical situations, you should choose the **single most likely option** according to the instruction.
- It is possible for one option to be the answer to more than one of the clinical situations.
- Marks will not be deducted for a wrong answer. Equally, you will not gain a mark if you mark more than one option.
- Only answers that are clearly struck horizontally across the correct response will guarantee a mark.
- Faint marking may be misread. All scores within 5 marks of the pass mark will be scrutinized.

Practice Paper 4: Part 2 – EMQs in Clinical Problem Solving

Theme: Tumour markers

Options
A Carcinoembryonic antigen
B Alpha-fetoprotein
C CA 19-9
D Human chorionic gonadotrophin
E CA 125
F Calcitonin
G Thyroglobulin
H Prostate-specific antigen

For each of the tumours below, select the most appropriate serum marker from the list of options above. Each option may be used once, more than once or not at all.

1. Testicular teratoma.
2. Papillary thyroid cancer.
3. Carcinoma of the pancreas.
4. Hepatocellular carcinoma.
5. Medullary thyroid cancer.
6. Ovarian adenocarcinoma.

Theme: Mass in the right iliac fossa (RIF)

Options
A Ectopic kidney
B Lymphoma
C Caecal carcinoma
D Ulcerative colitis
E Crohn's disease
F Tuberculosis
G Appendix mass
H Spigelian hernia

For each of the patients below, select the single most likely diagnosis from the list of options above. Each option may be used once, more than once or not at all.

7. A 30-year-old man is found to have a mobile mass and a scar in the RIF during a routine health check.
8. An 85-year-old woman presents with tiredness, weight loss and a mass in the RIF.
9. A 22-year-old Somali man presents with a 2-month history of weight loss, fever, night sweats and a mass in the RIF (Hb 10 g/dl; ESR 90).
10. A 15-year-old boy presents with a 2-week history of pain in the RIF. His family doctor started him on antibiotics 12 days ago. On examination, he was pyrexial with a mass in the RIF. He was previously fit and well.
11. A 20-year-old man presents with weight loss, fever, night sweats, itching and a mass in the RIF. Pain in the abdomen frequently followed drinking alcohol.
12. A 28-year-old man presents with RIF pain and diarrhoea that has worsened over a 3-week period. On examination, he has a mass in the RIF. Contrast follow-through shows the 'string sign of Cantor'.

Theme: Haematuria

Options
A Urinary tract infection
B Renal adenocarcinoma
C Transitional cell carcinoma of the bladder
D Benign prostatic hyperplasia
E Prostatic carcinoma
F Ureteric calculus

For each of the patients below, select the single most likely diagnosis from the list of options above. Each option may be used once, more than once or not at all.

13. A 40-year-old surgeon presents with a sudden onset of severe flank pain, nausea and vomiting. Urine microscopy confirmed the presence of microscopic haematuria.

14. A 25-year-old woman presents with burning dysuria, frequency and lower abdominal pain. Urinalysis showed microscopic haematuria.
15. A 75-year-old man presents with several months of backache, nocturia and frank haematuria. Sclerotic areas were seen on pelvic X-ray.
16. A 60-year-old man presents with a 2-month history of microscopic haematuria and right flank pain. Chest X-ray showed several opacities throughout the lung fields.
17. A 58-year-old female tyre factory worker presents with painless frank haematuria. Urine microscopy showed red cells, but no white cells.
18. A 70-year-old man presents with a progressive history of worsening frequency and nocturia and dribbling over the last 5 years. Rectal examination reveals an enlarged, smooth prostate.

Theme: Bone pain

Options

A Skeletal metastases
B Osteosarcoma
C Myeloma
D Primary hyperparathyroidism
E Tuberculosis
F Ewing sarcoma
G Paget's disease
H Osteomyelitis

For each of the patients below, select the single most likely diagnosis from the list of options above. Each option may be used once, more than once or not at all.

19. A 75-year-old man presents with dysuria, frequency and backache. X-rays showed multiple sclerotic areas in the lumbosacral spine.
20. A 10-year-old girl presents with a 2-week history of right shin pain and pyrexia. She was tender in this area. The white cell count and ESR were elevated.
21. A 50-year-old woman presents with backache and anaemia. X-rays showed lytic lesions in the skull and spine. ESR was elevated.
22. A 15-year-old girl presents with a painful swelling around the left knee. X-rays showed a lytic lesion with sun-ray spicules.
23. A 60-year-old woman presents with backache and abdominal pains. Plain X-rays showed osteoporosis, bone cysts and subperiosteal bone resorption.
24. A 60-year old man presents with hip pain. On examination, he is found to have a bowed femur and pain on movement of his hip. X-rays showed a motheaten pattern of the femur and pelvis, and blood tests showed a markedly elevated alkaline phosphatase.

Theme: Acid/base balance

Options
A Metabolic acidosis
B Metabolic alkalosis
C Respiratory acidosis
D Respiratory alkalosis

For each of the scenarios below, select the single most likely diagnosis from the list of options above. Each option may be used once, more than once or not at all.

25. A man who has vigorously exercised.
26. An anaemic woman at high altitude.
27. A patient with Guillain–Barré disease.
28. A patient with Conn syndrome.
29. A patient with a small-bowel fistula.
30. An extremely anxious 20-year-old woman who is needle-phobic and requires a blood test in clinic. She starts to feel faint after 10 minutes.

Theme: Blood constituents and their replacement

Options
A Whole blood
B Packed red cells
C Granulocyte concentrates
D Platelet concentrates
E Fresh-frozen plasma
F Human albumin 20%
G Cryoprecipitate
H Immunoglobulin

For each of the scenarios below, select the single most useful replacement fluid from the list of options above. Each option may be used once, more than once or not at all.

31. A patient at the end of an emergency abdominal aortic aneurysm repair who has already received 10 units of blood, but continues to bleed slowly from various areas. FBC: Hb 11.2 ; WBC 5.5; platelets 160.
32. A 75-year-old man who had a gastrectomy 2 days previously. Systolic blood pressure is 140 mmHg. Hb 7.6.
33. A patient with a haemarthrosis and von Willebrand's disease. Blood tests show impaired clotting function.
34. A 30-year-old woman with immune thrombocytopenia. Platelet count 50.
35. A 20-year-old man who had been stabbed in the epigastrium 10 minutes earlier, who was bleeding from the abdominal wound and vomiting copious amounts of blood. He was pale and semi-conscious, with a blood pressure of 65/40 mmHg.

36. A 40-year-old woman with immune thrombocytopenia presents with a haemarthrosis. Her platelet count is 10.

Theme: Skin ulcers

Options

A Venous ulcer
B Arterial ulcer
C Marjolin's ulcer
D Diabetic ulcer
E Neuropathic ulcer
F Pyoderma gangrenosum ulcer
G Syphilitic ulcer
H Tropical ulcer

For each of the scenarios below, select the single most likely diagnosis from the list of options above. Each option may be used once, more than once or not at all.

37. A patient with ulcerative colitis presenting with a painful large necrotic ulcer on the calf that started 2 weeks previously as several pustules that coalesced.
38. An 80-year old female non-smoker with a 3-month history of a 3 cm medial malleolus ulcer with sloping edges. The surrounding skin was brownish in colour.
39. A 25-year-old female who cut her leg 6 weeks ago on coral whilst scuba-diving presents with an enlarging non-healing painful wound on her calf.
40. A 70-year-old woman who had been treated for a static gaiter ulcer for 5 years developed a nodule at one side of the ulcer over 2 months, which started to bleed intermittently and then ulcerate itself.
41. A 40-year-old man in a wheelchair presented with a 2 cm ulcer over his heel. He had good pulses in both feet and the rest of the skin of his legs appeared normal.
42. A 70-year-old male smoker presented with a 2-week history of pain in his left foot, especially at night. On examination, he had a pale foot with an ulcer between his 4th and 5th toes. Pedal pulses were not palpable.

Theme: Principles of cancer treatment

Options

A Surgical excision
B Chemotherapy
C Neoadjuvant chemotherapy
D Hormonal therapy
E Radiotherapy
F Monoclonal antibody treatment
G No treatment

For each of the scenarios below, select the most appropriate initial treatment from the list of options above. Each option may be used once, more than once or not at all.

43. A 50-year-old previously fit woman presents with a 10 cm fixed breast mass with peau d'orange and enlarged ipsilateral axillary nodes. Core biopsy confirms a grade III inflammatory cancer.
44. A 45-year-old man presents with a bleeding polypoid mass at the anal margin. There are no palpable lymph nodes. Biopsy shows a squamous cell carcinoma.
45. A 30-year-old man presents with a 2 cm groin lump, weight loss and night sweats. Histology shows Reed–Sternberg cells.
46. A 55-year-old woman with her third recurrence of breast cancer, now involving her lumbar spine and ribs. She is relatively pain-free, but feels tired and is losing weight. Her original histology showed that the tumour was ER- and PR-negative, but HER2 strongly positive. She previously had two different types of combination chemotherapy with moderate response.
47. A 70-year-old man presents with hepatomegaly and back pain. Blood tests showed anaemia and a significantly elevated PSA.
48. An 80-year-old woman who lives alone presents with a 3 cm bleeding erythematous crusty lesion on her proximal thigh. Punch biopsy confirms a squamous cell carcinoma. She lives a long way from the nearest hospital.

Theme: Treatment of vascular disease

Options

A Balloon angioplasty
B Synthetic bypass
C Vein-graft bypass
D Conservative management only
E Embolectomy
F Endarterectomy
G Replacement of vessel with synthetic graft
H Amputation
I Stenting

For each of the scenarios below, select the most appropriate treatment from the list of options above. Each option may be used once, more than once or not at all.

49. A 65-year-old man developed several small patches of purplish skin over his left foot. Examination showed he had an easily palpable (and visible) aortic pulsation. Abdominal ultrasound showed that the aorta measured 6.7 cm in diameter.
50. A 60-year-old woman with ischaemic heart disease had a transient ischaemic attack causing temporary right-sided paralysis lasting 10 hours. CT scanning of her brain was normal. Carotid duplex showed a 60% stenosis of the left internal carotid.
51. A 60-year-old man presented with rest pain after previously experiencing claudication for the last 2 years. He was on maximal medical therapy. Angiograms showed an occlusion of the entire right superficial femoral artery. Distally, the only patent vessel was the anterior tibial at the level of the ankle, with good vessels in the foot. He was otherwise fit and well, with a good quality of life.
52. A 70-year-old woman with no previous peripheral vascular problems presented with a 4-hour history of a painful right leg. On examination, she was in atrial fibrillation and her right leg was cold and pale from the mid-tibia downwards. She had bilateral femoral pulses, but no other pulses on the right leg. All left-leg pulses were present. The right leg had reduced sensation and power.
53. A 60-year-old postman who had claudication at 50 yards could not work because of his symptoms. Angiography showed a right superficial femoral artery 95% stenosis, with good vessels proximally and distally. He was keen to return to work as soon as possible.
54. A 68-year-old man is feeling systemically unwell, 3 weeks after an elective abdominal aortic aneurysm repair. He is subsequently found to have an infected graft, which requires removal and a suitable revascularization procedure of the lower limbs.

Theme: Endocrine tumours

Options

A Parathyroid hyperplasia
B Medullary thyroid cancer
C Phaeochromocytoma
D Carcinoid syndrome
E Multiple endocrine neoplasia (MEN) type 1 syndrome
F Multiple endocrine neoplasia (MEN) type 2 syndrome
G Parathyroid adenoma

For each of the patients described below, select the most appropriate diagnosis from the list of options above. Each option may be used once, more than once or not at all.

55. A 65-year-old woman presents with joint stiffness, constipation and muscle weakness. Plain X-rays reveal a right renal calculus and evidence of osteitis fibrosa cystica.
56. A 42-year-old man presents with intermittent facial flushing, colicky abdominal pain and wheezing. Urinary 5-hydroxyindoleacetic acid levels are elevated.
57. A 24-year-old woman presents with hypercalcaemia and bilateral milky nipple discharge, but she has never been pregnant. PTH is elevated. Further hormone tests are awaited.
58. A 36-year-old man presents with raised blood pressure, tachycardia and excessive sweating. 24-hour urinary VMA is elevated.
59. A 42-year-old woman presents with a goitre and hypercalcaemia. 3 years previously, she had undergone a right adrenalectomy. Tests show an elevated PTH and calcitonin.
60. A 60-year-old woman presents with hypercalcaemia. A subsequent sestamibi scan shows four hot spots within the neck.

Theme: Gastrointestinal haemorrhage

Options

A Contrast enema
B Selective angiography
C Barium meal and follow-through
D Red blood cell scan
E Upper gastrointestinal (GI) endoscopy
F Colonoscopy

For each of the case scenarios described below, select the most suitable diagnostic and/or therapeutic investigation from the list of options above. Each option may be used once, more than once or not at all.

61. A 22-year-old woman with a strong family history of colorectal cancer presents with a positive faecal occult blood test.
62. An 80-year-old woman who had surgery for a fractured neck of the femur 1 week previously presents with painless abdominal distension and absolute constipation for 5 days. She also has chronic airways disease. Prior to admission, her bowel habit was normal. On examination, her abdomen was tympanitic, non-tender and silent, with no masses. Rectal examination showed haemorrhoids and fresh blood on the glove. Abdominal X-rays showed dilated large-bowel loops.
63. A 55-year-old man presents to casualty with melaena, pallor and dizziness.
64. A 65-year-old woman with aortic stenosis presents with mixed dark and bright red rectal bleeding with clots. Her pulse was 110 bpm and her blood pressure 90/60. Rigid sigmoidoscopy had to be abandoned due to poor vision in view of the amount of blood/clot in the lumen. It was thought that colonoscopy would be similarly difficult.
65. A 35-year-old man presents with chronic anaemia and positive faecal occult blood tests. Examination is normal apart from bluish pigmented lesions on his lips, which had been present for many years. He had previously undergone an OGD and colonoscopy 3 months beforehand.

Theme: Pancreatic and hepatobiliary disease

Options

A Gallstone in the common bile duct
B Mirizzi syndrome
C Chronic pancreatitis
D Acute pancreatitis
E Carcinoma of the head of the pancreas
F Cholangiocarcinoma
G Sclerosing cholangitis
H Primary biliary cirrhosis
I Hepatocellular carcinoma
J Ascending cholangitis

For each of the patients described below, select the most likely diagnosis from the list of options above. Each option can be used once, more than once or not at all.

66. A 70-year old ex-alcoholic man presents with intermittent upper abdominal pain for at least 9 months. He was recently diagnosed with diabetes and his stools have become paler and greasy. CT scans show inflammation with a few flecks of calcification around the pancreas region, and ERCP was normal.
67. A 40-year-old woman presents with nausea, fever and epigastric pain radiating to the back. She is jaundiced, but there is no abdominal tenderness. She has recently had a laparoscopic cholecystecomy. Blood tests show a bilirubin of 92 μmol/l and a white cell count of 18. Ultrasound shows a dilated common bile duct.
68. A 38-year-old woman presents with epigastric pain radiating round to her back, fever and vomiting. She is pyrexial, with guarding over the right hypochondrium. Blood tests show a white cell count of 16 and bilirubin of 75 μmol/l. Ultrasound shows a dilated common hepatic duct but a normal common bile duct and a thickened gallbladder wall.
69. A 78-year-old man presents with a 6-month history of epigastric and back pain associated with significant weight loss. On examination, he is cachectic and jaundiced and has a palpable gallbladder.
70. A 60-year-old man with a past history of ulcerative colitis presents with painless jaundice. Subsequent ERCP shows widespread irregular narrowing of his biliary system. Biopsies and biliary washings exclude carcinoma.
71. A 55-year-old African man presents with a 4-month history and weight loss. He is a known carrier of hepatitis C. On examination, he has hepatomegaly. Blood tests show elevated alpha-fetoprotein and deranged liver function tests.

Theme: Anaesthetic techniques

Options

A Local anaesthesia
B Regional nerve block
C Epidural and spinal anaesthesia
D General anaesthesia

For each of the scenarios described below, select the most suitable choice of anaesthesia from the list of options above. Each option can be used once, more than once or not at all.

72. An 80-year-old man with significant cardiorespiratory problems who requires an above-knee amputation for gangrene of the lower limb.
73. A 20-year-old fit, healthy and sensible woman who is due to undergo removal of a 2 cm fibroadenoma of the breast.
74. A 50-year-old fit and healthy man who presents to casualty with a strangulated inguinal hernia that requires emergency surgical repair.
75. A 30-year-old woman who has been booked to undergo an elective caesarian section for her second child.
76. A 65-year-old woman who sustained a Colles fracture that requires manipulation before the application of a forearm plaster.

Theme: Rectal bleeding

Options
A Haemorrhoids
B Acute anal fissure
C Ulcerative colitis
D Crohn's disease
E Familial adenomatous polyposis
F Squamous cell carcinoma
G Thrombosed perianal varix
H Adenocarcinoma of the colon
I Ischaemic colitis
J Rectal prolapse

For each of the patients described below, select the most likely diagnosis from the list of options above. Each option can be used once, more than once or not at all.

77. A 70-year-old man presented with the painless passage of mixed dark and bright red rectal bleeding. He had, however, experienced severe abdominal pains the preceding day, which had now settled. Apart from ischaemic heart disease, he was otherwise healthy. Contrast enema revealed a smooth stricture in the region of the splenic flexure and proximal descending colon.
78. A 25-year-old man presented with copious bloody diarrhoea. Stool cultures were negative. Colonoscopy showed an inflamed mucosa from the anal margin to the mid-descending colon. In later years, he underwent a colectomy.
79. A 75-year-old woman presented with a 4-month history of intermittent perianal bleeding and continual soreness. Examination showed a friable lesion on one side of the anal verge and palpable inguinal lymph nodes.
80. An 18-year-old man with a family history of bowel cancer presented with fresh rectal bleeding. Sigmoidoscopy revealed multiple (>100) rectal polyps, some of which were biopsied.
81. A 20-year-old man presented with a 5-day history of sharp pain on defaecation, associated with bright red blood on the toilet paper. Rectal examination showed the presence of a 'sentinel pile'.
82. A 78-year-old man presented with weight loss, irregular bowel habit and passage of mixed dark/bright red blood rectally. Contrast enema showed an irregular stricture of the left colon.

Theme: Breast cancer treatment

Options

A Modified radical mastectomy
B Wide local excision and axillary clearance
C Simple mastectomy
D Postoperative radiotherapy and tamoxifen
E Postoperative chemotherapy, radiotherapy and tamoxifen
F Postoperative chemotherapy and LHRH analogues
G Postoperative radiotherapy and aromatase inhibitors
H Radiotherapy alone
I Neoadjuvant chemotherapy

For each of the patients described below, select the most likely single treatment from the list of options above. Each option can be used once, more than once or not at all.

83. A 58-year-old woman presents with a 6 cm mass in the outer half of her right breast. Mammograms and core biopsy confirm an invasive lobular cancer. She is booked for surgery.
84. A 50-year-old woman presents with a 2 cm cancer in the left breast. She undergoes wide excision and axillary dissection. Histology shows a 2.5 cm invasive ductal carcinoma with clear margins. It is ER-positive. 4 out of 12 lymph nodes contain tumour.
85. A 52-year-old woman undergoes breast screening, which shows a small area of microcalcification in the right upper inner quadrant. Nothing is palpable. Core biopsy reveals ductal carcinoma in situ (DCIS). Excision biopsy of the area shows 16 mm of high-grade DCIS, which has been widely excised (>1 cm).
86. A 33-year-old woman presents with a 5 cm breast lump, which after core biopsy is found to be a grade 3 invasive ductal carcinoma. She is keen to preserve her breast and avoid mastectomy.
87. A 75-year-old woman underwent a breast-conserving procedure and sentinel node biopsy and was found to have a 3 cm grade 2 node-negative invasive ductal carcinoma. The tumour was ER-positive. Margins were clear. She had a past history of DVTs and angina.
88. A 60-year old woman presents with a 2 cm lump in the upper outer quadrant of the right breast. She was otherwise fit and healthy. Core biopsy confirms an invasive ductal carcinoma.

Theme: The Glasgow Coma Score

Options
A 3
B 4
C 6
D 7
E 8
F 9
G 10
H 12
I 13
J 14
K 15

For each of the clinical scenarios described below, select the Glasgow Coma Score from the list of options above. Each option can be used once, more than once or not at all.

89. A patient who withdraws and opens her eyes to a painful stimulus, but does not utter any sounds.
90. A man who abnormally flexes to a painful stimulus, but does not open his eyes. He utters incomprehensible sounds.
91. A drowsy patient who opens his eyes to speech and localizes pain, but utters a confused conversation.
92. A patient with diffuse axonal injury who has no motor response to painful stimuli and keeps his eyes closed at all times. He is not able to make any sounds.
93. A woman following a car accident who elicits an extensor response to pain, but does not make sounds or open her eyes.
94. A 22-year-old man who had been drinking alcohol and became involved in an altercation presented with bruising and lacerations to his face and forehead. He was initially asleep but opened his eyes on being questioned. He then spoke in a confused manner, but obeyed commands.

Theme: Preoperative investigations

Options

A None required
B Full blood count and urea and electrolytes (FBC and U&Es)
C FBC, U&Es, chest X-ray and electrocardiogram (ECG)
D FBC, U&Es, group and save (G&S), chest X-ray and ECG
E All routine bloods, chest X-ray, ECG and echocardiogram
F All routine bloods, chest X-ray, ECG, spirometry and blood gases

For each of the patients described below, select the most appropriate single group of preoperative investigations from the list of options above. Each option can be used once, more than once or not at all.

95. A 65-year-old woman undergoing a femoro–distal bypass who had previously undergone an aortic valve replacement 3 years earlier.
96. A 70-year-old lifelong smoker undergoing an elective laparotomy for colonic cancer who requires daily inhalers.
97. A 20-year-old fit man undergoing a day-case inguinal hernia repair under general anaesthesia.
98. A 40-year-old, previously fit woman undergoing a cystoscopy for unexplained haematuria.
99. A 65-year-old smoker due to have a modified radical mastectomy for breast cancer.
100. A 65-year-old previously healthy lifelong smoker undergoing manipulation of an ankle fracture under general anaesthesia.

Theme: The acute abdomen

Options

A Acute diverticulitis
B Acute pancreatitis
C Acute cholecystitis
D Small-bowel obstruction
E Large-bowel obstruction
F Acute mesenteric ischaemia
G Perforated duodenal ulcer
H Acute cholecystitis
I Ruptured abdominal aortic aneurysm
J Acute appendicitis

For each of the patients described below, select the most appropriate single group of preoperative investigations from the list of options above. Each option can be used once, more than once or not at all.

101. A 55-year-old man presented to the casualty department with a 2-day history of severe pain in the epigastric area radiating to the back. He was also vomiting. On examination, he was tachycardic, tachypnoeic, hypotensive (95/40 mmHg) and had a tender non-pulsatile mass in the upper abdomen. There was periumbilical bruising.
102. A 70-year-old woman with a longstanding history of ischaemic heart disease presented with a sudden onset of severe generalized abdominal pain. She vomited twice. She opened her bowels earlier. On examination, she was in atrial fibrillation and hypotensive (100/50 mmHg), with a diffusely tender abdomen but no consistent guarding or palpable masses. Her Hb was 13 g/dl, WCC 23 000/mm^3 and amylase 200 units. Abdominal and chest X-rays were unremarkable.
103. A 68-year old woman smoker presented as an emergency with a 5-day history of lower abdominal pain that had significantly increased over the last 24 hours. Her bowels had been irregular for 2 years. She had two abdominal scars. On examination, she was pyrexial, with a tender mass over the left lower quadrant. Rectal examination was normal.
104. A 25-year-old presented via emergency with a 3-hour history of generalized severe abdominal pain, associated with vomiting. On examination, his virgin abdomen was rigid and tender throughout, with absent bowel sounds. In addition, he was tachypnoeic and tachycardic. Initial routine blood tests were normal.

105. A 77-year-old smoker presented with a 4-hour history of severe back pain and collapse. He had never had any previous surgery, although he was on medication for angina and diabetes. On examination, he was obese, pale, tachycardic (120 sinus rhythm) and hypotensive (90/60 mmHg), and becoming confused. He was tender mainly in the periumbilical and epigastric areas. Subsequent CT scan showed no free intra-abdominal air.

106. A 70-year-old woman presented with a 5-day history of progressive intermittent abdominal pain and absolute constipation. Examination revealed a tympanitic distended abdomen, with tenderness in the right iliac fossa with guarding. Bowel sounds were high-pitched.

Theme: Medicine and the law

Options

A Expert witness
B Doctor who attended the patient during the previous week
C Doctor who has practised for at least 5 years
D Coroner
E Registrar of Births and Deaths
F Any medically qualified doctor

From the list of options above, select the most appropriate person to perform the following tasks:

107. Certify a patient death.
108. Complete Part 2 of the death certificate.
109. Call an inquest.
110. Give information to a court judge as to whether negligence may have been caused by another doctor.
111. Send information regarding causation of death to the Office of Population Censuses and Surveys (OPCS).

Theme: The painful swollen knee

Options

A Tibial plateau fracture
B Fracture of the patella
C Anterior cruciate ligament injury
D Collateral ligament injury
E Rheumatoid arthritis
F Osteoarthritis
G Gout
H Meniscal tear

For each of the patients described below, select the most appropriate single diagnosis from the list of options above. Each option can be used once, more than once or not at all.

112. A 30-year-old footballer presents with sudden pain of his right knee after twisting his leg in a football match. Needle aspiration of the knee reveals blood and he has a positive anterior draw sign.
113. A 75-year-old obese woman presents with a 6-week history of progressive knee swelling and pain. Examination shows an effusion and limited flexion with crepitus.
114. A 35-year-old rugby player is knocked over from the side and sustains a painful swollen left knee immediately afterwards. On examination, he is tender along the medial joint line, with pain and apprehension on attempted abduction of the leg with respect to the knee.
115. A 35-year-old hockey player presents with a 2-month history of intermittent pain of her right knee on exercise, which occasionally locks. Arthroscopy shows a parrot's beak lesion.
116. A 70-year-old woman presents with a painful swollen right knee after falling directly onto the knee. She is subsequently unable to extend the knee. Aspiration of the joint shows blood and fat globules. The injury is repaired by means of wires.
117. A 60-year-old overweight man presents with a 7-day history of a progressively painful left knee. He denies any trauma or any other joint problems. Examination shows a swollen red knee. Effusion fluid is diagnostic.

Theme: Clinical examination tests

Options

A Simmond's test
B McMurray's test
C Chovstek's test/sign
D Caloric test
E Allen's test
F Trendelenberg's test
G Ortolani's test
H Buerger's test
I Apprehension test
J Homan's test/sign

For each of the clinical situations described below, select the most appropriate clinical examination test from the list of options above. Each option can be used once, more than once or not at all.

118. A patient who describes circumoral tingling 24 hours after a parathyroidectomy.
119. A 35-year-old man who presents with sudden onset of pain over the back of the lower right leg during a squash match. He felt as though something had hit the back of his leg.
120. A 6-week-old boy undergoing a routine postnatal check for abnormalities.
121. A 40-year-old footballer who injured his knee and is suspected of having a meniscal tear.
122. A 70-year-old woman who has calf pain 10 days after a right hemicolectomy for cancer.
123. A 65-year-old patient who was admitted for three-vessel coronary artery surgery. The surgeon planned to use the the left internal mammary artery, left radial artery and saphenous vein for the grafts.

Theme: Anorectal surgery

Options

A No treatment
B Oral laxatives only
C Topical GTN cream
D Rest, ice packs, topical local anaesthetics and laxatives
E Injection sclerotherapy/banding
F Milligan–Morgan operation
G Anal stretch
H Lateral sphincterotomy

For each of the patients described below, select the most appropriate treatment from the list of options above. Each option can be used once, more than once or not at all.

124. A 32-week pregnant woman presents with large prolapsed piles that are extremely painful and not reducible by the patient.
125. A 20-year-old man presents with sharp anal pain and fresh blood on defaecation, which has not settled after 3 weeks of laxatives.
126. A 45-year-old woman presents with intermittent bright red rectal bleeding and prolapsed swellings that reduce spontaneously after defaecation. Proctoscopy confirms the presence of moderate-sized haemorrhoids.
127. A 25-year-old man presents with a 24-hour history of a painful lump suddenly appearing around his anal margin when straining. He denies any bleeding. Examination confirms the presence of a 1 cm hemispherical purplish swelling on the anal verge that is exquisitely tender and partly fluctuant.
128. A 65-year-old fit man presents with permanently prolapsed large haemorrhoids that have been present for many years. He would like treatment because of the mucus soiling his underclothes.
129. A 23-year-old man presents with sharp anal pain and fresh blood on defaecation that has not settled after a period of topical anal treatment, which was also causing headaches.

Theme: Surgical sutures

Options

A 6/0 nylon
B 4/0 PDS
C 2/0 Vicryl
D 2/0 silk
E 3/0 nylon
F 1 loop PDS
G 1 nylon deep tension sutures
H Clips

For each of the situations described below, select the most appropriate suture from the list of options above. Each option can be used once, more than once or not at all.

130. A suction drain following laparoscopic cholecystectomy requires suturing in place.
131. A 3 cm traumatic scalp laceration over the vertex requires closure.
132. A breast wound from which a fibroadenoma has just been excised.
133. Repair of the external oblique aponeurosis during hernia repair.
134. Closure of a dehisced abdomen in a sick patient on steroids with low serum albumin.
135. Suturing of a blepharoplasty.

Theme: Visual field defects

Options

A Ipsilateral mononuclear field loss
B Lower homonymous quadrantanopia
C Upper homonymous quadrantanopia
D Ipsilateral homonymous hemianopia
E Contralateral homonymous hemianopia
F Bitemporal hemianopia

For the brain/nerve lesions described below, select the most appropriate resulting visual field defect from the list of options given above. Each option may be used once, more than once or not at all.

136. Optic nerve injury.
137. Optic chiasma injury.
138. Temporal lobe injury.
139. Unilateral occipital lobe injury.
140. Parietal lobe injury.

Theme: Structures damaged during surgery

Options
A Ilioinguinal nerve
B Genitofemoral nerve
C Recurrent laryngeal nerve
D External laryngeal nerve
E Femoral nerve
F Obturator nerve
G Sciatic nerve
H Hypoglossal nerve
I Lingual nerve
J Marginal mandibular nerve
K Phrenic nerve

For each of the procedures described below, select the most appropriate nerve that may be damaged from the list of options given above. Each option may be used once, more than once or not at all.

141. Total hip replacement.
142. Lichtenstein repair.
143. Ligating the superior thyroid artery during a thyroidectomy.
144. The surgical approach for excision of a submandibular gland tumour.
145. Excision of an inferior parathyroid gland.

Theme: Lower-limb trauma

Options
A Skeletal traction
B Intramedullary nail
C Plate and screws
D External fixator
E Plaster of Paris
F Above-knee amputation
G Below-knee amputation

For each of the clinical scenarios described below, select the single most appropriate treatment from the list of options given above. Each option may be used once, more than once or not at all.

146. A 60-year-old man is knocked from his motorbike. He sustains a comminuted Gustillo 3c fracture of his tibia. The tibial nerve is transected.
147. A 40-year-old woman has a closed spiral fracture of the lower third of the tibia. The ankle joint appears to be unaffected.
148. A 30-year-old man is hit by a car bumper. He has a closed transverse fracture of the midshaft of both the tibia and the fibula.

149. A 25-year-old man sustains an injury during a game of football. X-ray shows a displaced Weber B fracture of the fibula associated with a fracture of the medial maleolus.

150. A 25-year-old man is involved in a road traffic accident. He has a highly comminuted fracture of both the tibia and the fibula. There is a large area of skin loss over the fracture that will require plastic surgery input. The foot is neurovascularly intact.

Answers

Practice Paper 1: Answers

1. Answers

A True
B True
C False
D True
E False

2. Answers

A False
B True
C True
D True
E True

The lipopolysaccharide portion of the cell wall of Gram-negative bacteria is an example of an endotoxin. Most exotoxins are polypeptides; examples are tetanus toxoid and botulinum toxin. Most exotoxins are destroyed at 60 °C, whereas endotoxins are stable at 100 °C.

3. Answers

A True
B False
C True
D True
E False

Pulse and spinal reflexes are irrelevant. The six tests are fixed pupils, absent corneal reflex, absent vestibulo-ocular reflexes, no motor responses of face or limbs after supra-orbital pressure, absent gag reflex and absent respiratory effort with stimulation of the respiratory centre by raising $PaCO_2$ to $>$ 6.65 kPa.

4. Answers

A True
B True
C True
D False
E True

Clostridium tetani causes tetanus. *C. difficile* causes pseudomembranous colitis. *C. perfringens* causes gas gangrene. *C. botulinum* causes botulism food poisoning. Anthrax is caused by a *Bacillus*.

5. Answers

A False
B True
C True
D False
E True

The long thoracic nerve arises from C5, C6 and C7. It supplies the serratus anterior muscle whilst the thoracodorsal nerve supplies the latissimus dorsi muscle. The posterior wall of the axilla is made up of the latissimus dorsi muscle (thoracodorsal nerve), subscapularis muscle (subscapular nerve) and the teres major muscle (lower subscapular nerve).

6. Answers

A False
B False
C False
D True
E True

Parotid pleomorphic adenomas are the commonest salivary gland tumours. They do not have a true capsule – hence the possibility of recurrence, even though they are considered benign. Surgery is the treatment of choice. Facial nerve palsy is commoner in malignant tumours, but does rarely occur in pleomorphic adenomas as well.

7. Answers

A False
B True
C False
D False
E True

The quadrangular space is bounded by the teres major muscle inferiorly and the teres minor muscle superiorly. The subscapularis tendon inserts into the lesser tuberosity of the humerus. The axillary nerve is at risk of damage in humeral neck fractures.

8. Answers

A True
B False
C True
D True
E True

The carpal tunnel (formed by the flexor retinaculum over the eight carpal bones) contains the four tendons of the flexor digitorum superficialis (FDS), four tendons of the flexor digitorum profundus (FDP), flexor policis longus (FPL) and flexor carpi radialis (FCR), and the median nerve. The radial artery passes through the anatomical snuff-box.

9. Answers

A True
B False
C True
D False
E False

There are many causes of SIRS, including trauma and sepsis. There is an increased output of insulin, steroids and catecholamines. Other than the white count, a core temperature of $>38°C$ or $<36°C$, heart rate >90 bpm, and respiratory rate of >20 breaths/min may be used to diagnose SIRS. Nitric oxide (NO), not nitrous oxide (N_2O), may be used in SIRS.

10. Answers

A True
B False
C True
D False
E True

The intra-aortic balloon pump is a device used to boost a low blood pressure in times of cardiogenic shock. It is inflated in diastole and deflated in systole. It increases the diastolic pressure, thus increasing the mean arterial pressure (MAP = diastolic BP + 1/3 pulse pressure). It is contraindicated in severe aortic regurgitation, as the '2nd pump' in diastole would force blood back into an already dilated left ventricle.

11. Answers

A False
B False
C True
D True
E False

Bleeding is usually from Little's area, a plexus of vessels on the anterior aspect of the nasal septum. Pressure over the lower nose may compress a low bleeding vessel. Pressure over the bony part of the nose is useless. Silver nitrate or diathermy can be used to cauterize visible bleeders. Bleeding from further back can be tamponaded with a Foley catheter inflated in the postnasal space with or without insertion of an anterior pack. Ligation of the *external* carotid artery may be necessary.

12. Answers

A False
B True
C True
D True
E True

The scaphoid articulates with the lunate, trapezoid, trapezium, capitate and radius. It is palpable in the anatomical snuff-box, with the radial artery running over it. The bone has a precarious blood supply from a distal origin; therefore a fracture through the waist of the scaphoid may cause proximal necrosis. The flexor retinaculum attaches between the tubercle of the scaphoid and the trapezium on the radial side and the hook of the hamate and the pisiform on the ulnar side.

13. Answers

A True
B False
C False
D False
E False

Neither osteoporosis nor Paget's disease cause hypercalcaemia, although they are both diseases of the bones. Secondary hyperparathyroidism is the parathyroid glands' response to hypocalcaemia. Primary and tertiary hyperparathyroidism both cause hypercalcaemia. Pancreatitis may be caused by hypercalcaemia, but can also cause hypocalcaemia.

14. Answers

A True
B False
C True
D False
E True

ARDS is defined as pulmonary oedema of non-cardiac origin. It can be caused by direct lung injury (e.g. inhalation of smoke) or as part of the systemic inflammatory response syndrome. To make the diagnosis, the patient must have reduced gas exchange, characteristic chest X-ray appearance and a normal pulmonary capillary wedge pressure, thus excluding cardiogenic pulmonary oedema. It carries a poor prognosis.

15. Answers

A False
B True
C True
D True
E True

The epiploic foramen (of Winslow) is bounded anteriorly by the free edge of the lesser omentum, which contains the portal triad: the hepatic artery, the portal vein and the common bile duct. A finger in the epiploic foramen pinching the portal triad against a thumb anteriorly is the 'Pringle manoeuvre' and is useful to slow bleeding from the liver. The superior boundary is the caudate surface of the liver.

16. Answers

A True
B True
C False
D False
E True

Atraumatic handling of tissue decreases the load of necrotic or non-viable cells at the wound margin. Tensionless wound edge apposition reduces wound edge ischaemia and hypoxic injury. Meticulous hemostasis reduces the risk of haematoma formation and subsequent inflammation to clear the wound of blood. Deep sutures are best placed only into collagen-laden structures that will hold tension, i.e. fascia and dermis. Fat does not contain collagen and will not hold tension. Therefore, fatty tissue should not be sutured as a separate layer. Given that epithelialization of an incision is normally complete within 24–48 hours, there is no reason to protect the incision from water beyond this time period.

17. Answers

A True
B True
C True
D False
E False

Heparin-associated thrombocytopenia is a syndrome in which a heparin-dependent platelet antibody causes aggregation of platelets. Activation of platelets in this setting results in thrombocytopenia, thrombosis and embolic episodes. Antithrombin III deficiency accounts for about 2% of venous thrombotic events. Other hereditary thrombotic conditions are protein C deficiency, protein S deficiency and factor V Leiden mutation. von Willebrand's disease is a hereditary coagulation factor deficiency leading to prolonged bleeding time. It is caused by a reduction of factor VIII activity and the von Willebrand factor, which is an adhesive protein that mediates platelet adhesion to collagen. Severe vitamin C deficiency results in a disorder in soft tissue that increases vascular permeability and fragility, resulting in the potential for bleeding disorders.

18. Answers

A True
B True
C False
D True
E True

Hypoproteinaemia leads to diminution of fibroblast proliferation, proteoglycan and collagen synthesis, angiogenesis, and wound remodelling. Wound infection is the most important factor associated with the risk of wound failure. Although anaemia was once believed to be a significant cause of wound disruption, studies have shown that, in the absence of malnutrition or hypovolaemia, anaemia with a haematocrit greater than 15% does not interfere with wound healing. In contrast, molecular oxygen is critical for collagen synthesis. The role of age in collagen synthesis is not clear, but the incidence of wound failure and incisional hernias is greater in patients older than 60.

19. Answers

A True
B True
C True
D False
E True

Determinants of cerebral blood flow include arterial pCO_2 and pO_2, systemic arterial pressure, intracranial pressure and temperature. Factors that may affect intracranial pressure are head position, jugular venous obstruction and positive end-expiratory pressure. *Remember*: cerebral perfusion pressure = arterial blood pressure – intracranial pressure.

20. Answers

A False
B False
C True
D True
E False

Because local anaesthetics act from within the nerve, they work best in their non-ionized form as they must first cross the lipid bilayer of the membrane. They inhibit transmission of nerve impulses by reducing sodium membrane permeability and the displacement of ionized calcium. All local anesthetics consist of a hydrophilic region and a hydrophobic region separated by an alkyl chain. The bond of the alkyl chain is either an ester or an amide, and these drugs are classified based on this bond. All local anesthetics except cocaine produce vasodilatation and are weak bases.

21. Answers

A True
B False
C False
D True
E True

Markedly elevated serum calcium levels produce polydipsia, polyuria and thirst. Vigorous volume repletion and saline diuresis correct the extracellular fluid volume deficit and promote the urinary excretion of calcium. Metastatic breast cancer is the most common cause of hypercalcaemia. The calcitonin effect on calcium is diminished with repeated administrations.

22. Answers

A False
B True
C False
D True
E False

Follicular carcinoma is more common in older patients (peak incidence in the fifth decade). The tumor has a marked propensity for vascular invasion and spreads haematogenously to bone, lung, liver and central nervous system sites. Local nodal metastases are less common than in papillary carcinoma. Extensive angioinvasion indicates a less favorable prognosis. Papillary carcinoma is the most common type of well-differentiated thyroid carcinoma. Follicular carcinomas are rarely multicentric.

23. Answers

A True
B False
C True
D False
E False

Iodine is necessary for the synthesis of thyroid hormone, and approximately 200–500 mg is ingested daily. Most of it is absorbed from the small intestine and is cleared from the plasma by the thyroid gland. TSH is required for the normal production and secretion of thyroid hormone. TSH also has a major role in thyroid growth. The thyroid gland has a storage reserve of approximately 3 weeks. TRH is produced by the superoptic and paraventricular nuclei within the hypothalamus and passes down their axones. Following secretion into the hypophyseal portal blood systems, TRH passes to the pituitary and induces stimulation of TSH secretion. Mono-iodo*tyrosine* is combined with di-iodo*tyrosine* to produce tri-iodo*thyronine* (T_3).

24. Answers

A False
B False
C True
D False
E False

Although pharmaceutical agents are useful in preparing the patient for surgery or in palliating the patient with recurrent adrenal carcinoma, no agents render definitive therapy for adrenal tumours. The treatment of adrenal tumors is primarily surgical removal. Congenital adrenal hyperplasia stands alone among the primary, hyperfunctioning adrenal syndromes that are amenable to medical therapy for definitive treatment with cortisone acetate and possibly fludrocortisone. Cushing's disease is due to an ACTH-secreting pituitary adenoma, whereas Cushing syndrome may be due to any cause of raised levels of circulating corticosteroids.

25. Answers

A False
B True
C False
D False
E False

The parathyroid glands develop from the third and fourth pharyngeal pouches, along with the thymus. There are four glands in the vast majority of persons. Calcitonin is secreted by the medullary C cells of the thyroid. Vitamin D_3 hydroxylation occurs in the kidney.

26. Answers

A False
B True
C False
D False
E True

Medullary thyroid cancer and phaeochromocytoma occur in both MEN 2A and MEN 2B syndromes. Patients with MEN 2A may also develop hyperplasia of the parathyroid glands. Although some investigators have reported equivocal histological abnormalities in the parathyroid glands of patients with MEN 2B, hyperparathyroidism is not a component of this syndrome.

In contrast to patients with MEN 2A, those with MEN 2B have a characteristic phenotype, including a tall, thin 'marfanoid' habitus. Patients with MEN 2B also develop multiple neuromas on the lips, tongue and oral mucosa, creating the appearance of thick lips. Pituitary adenomas are part of the MEN type I syndrome.

27. Answers

A True
B True
C True
D True
E False

Common types of hyperthyroidism include diffuse toxic goitre (Graves' disease) and toxic adenoma or toxic multinodular goitre (Plummer's disease). Uncommon causes include functioning metastatic thyroid carcinoma, trophoblastic tumours that secrete human chorionic gonadotrophin (having thyroid-stimulating properties), inappropriate secretion of TSH by pituitary tumours, iodide-induced hyperfunction and thyroiditis.

28. Answers

A False
B False
C True
D False
E False

Hashimoto's disease is the best-known of the immunological thyroid diseases. It is the most common cause of goitrous hypothyroidism in adults and of sporadic goitre in children. The incidence is 0.3–1.5 cases per 1000 population per year and it is 10–15 times more common in women than in men, with the highest incidence in the group aged 30–50 years. Graves' disease characteristically causes hyperthyroidism. Riedel's thyroiditis (dense fibrosis of the thyroid) is very rare. de Quervain's thyroiditis (viral infection) is uncommon. Multinodular goitre patients are usually euthyroid.

29. Answers

A True
B False
C True
D True
E False

Head injuries cause the majority of deaths following road traffic accidents, with rupture of the thoracic aorta being the second most common cause of fatality. Head injury itself rarely produces hypotensive shock. It is only in the terminal phases of brain death that hypotension may be attributable to head injury alone. Therefore, hypotension in trauma patients must be assumed to be secondary to volume depletion or ongoing haemorrhage elsewhere. A rapid and complete neurological assessment is a crucial part of the initial assessment of all trauma patients. The ultimate outcome of a brain injury is dependent on adequate cerebral perfusion and oxygenation. *Constricted* pupils may be due to opiates.

30. Answers

A True
B True
C True
D True
E True

CEA is relatively non-specific, and each of the listed cancers can cause elevated levels.

31. Answers

A False
B True
C False
D False
E False

Approximately 40% of breast cancers have c-*erb*B-2 gene expression. Tumours that express c-*erb*B-2 have a poorer prognosis. Oestrogen receptor-positive tumours have a better prognosis, as they are usually ameniable to hormone manipulation therapy.

32. Answers

A False
B True
C True
D False
E True

In inherited retinoblastomas an abnormal *Rb* gene is transmitted to half the offspring. As long as a normal allele is present, the tumour does not develop, and the abnormal germline mutation behaves in a recessive fashion. However, a second mutation of the normal allele (somatic cell mutation) may occur in a retinal cell, leading to the development of the tumour. This is an example of tumour supressor gene loss. In sporadic retinoblastomas development of a tumour requires two somatic mutations. The genetic loss in retinoblastomas involves deletion of DNA from chromosome 13q.

33. Answers

A True
B False
C True
D True
E False

The Epstein–Barr virus (EBV), of the herpesvirus group, has been implicated in the aetiology of Burkitt lymphoma and nasopharyngeal carcinoma. Continued exposure to EBV results in high titres of antibody to the virus antigen and a 30-fold increase in risk of cancer compared with control populations. Human papillomavirus (HPV) is responsible for genital warts. Infected women have significantly increased risk for cervical carcinoma. Hepatitis B virus (HBV) is implicated in the aetiology of hepatocellular carcinoma.

34. Answers

A False
B True
C False
D True
E True

Occlusion of the common iliac artery is usually associated with claudication of the thigh and calf. Angiography should be done to establish the diagnosis and to assess the peripheral arterial system. Angiography is also quite helpful in deciding whether or not balloon angioplasty is indicated, since it can be used successfully in many patients. Collateral vessels are usually apparent on the angiogram.

35. Answers

A False
B True
C False
D True
E False

The portal vein provides three-quarters of the total hepatic blood flow, the hepatic artery one-quarter. The portal vein contains blood from the gut and is approximately 85% saturated with oxygen. The hepatic artery oxygen saturation is approximately 99%. However, each vessel supplies roughly equal amounts of oxygen to the liver. Whereas hepatic metastases often arrive there via the portal vein, most of their blood supply comes from the hepatic artery. The hepatic *vein* divides the liver into anatomical segments.

36. Answers

A True
B True
C True
D True
E False

Diathermy (monopolar) should not be used on appendages (e.g. penis) or isolated tissue (e.g. testis) because of the possible risk of damage to the blood supply/pedicle. The patient plate should be placed as close to the operative field as possible in order to reduce the amount of tissue through which the current passes.

37. Answers

A False
B False
C True
D True
E False

The most common cause of hyponatraemia is an excess of free water rather than a deficit of total body sodium. Hyponatraemia is frequently seen in postoperative or post-trauma patients because increased ADH secretion acts on the collecting tubules of the kidney to increase free-water reabsorption. Hyponatraemia most often results from excess free water. Most surgical patients with hyponatraemia are euvolaemic or hypervolaemic. Such patients, if asymptomatic, are best treated by free-water restriction. Hypernatraemia is a less common problem in surgical patients than hyponatraemia and is usually the result of excess free-water loss associated with hypovolaemia. The symptoms of hypernatraemia are related to the hyperosmolar state. CNS effects predominate because of cellular dehydration as water passes into the extracellular space. Prompt treatment of hypernatraemia is essential. But too rapid correction is associated with significant risk of cerebral oedema and herniation.

38. Answers

A False
B False
C True
D True
E False

The testicular arteries arise from the abdominal aorta near the renal arteries. The left testicular vein enters the left renal vein whereas the right testicular vein usually enters the inferior vena cava (note the increased incidence of left-sided varicocoele). The Leydig cells secrete testosterone, the Sertoli cells secrete inhibin. Each primary spermatocyte gives rise by the process of meiosis to two secondary spermatocytes, each of which divides by mitosis to produce two spermatids. These four spermatids then differentiate to form four spermatozoa. A patent processus vaginalis predisposes to *indirect* inguinal hernia formation.

39. Answers

A True
B True
C False
D True
E True

BPH can lead to acute or chronic urinary retention. The stagnant urine secondary to incomplete voiding predisposes to infection and stone formation. Bladder diverticulae arise after chronic obstruction. BPH does not predispose to prostate cancer, but the two often occur together. Renal failure and uraemia is the end-result of chronic bladder outflow obstruction.

40. Answers

A True
B True
C True
D False
E False

Above the arcuate line, the anterior rectus sheath is made up of the aponeuroses of the external oblique and half of the internal oblique muscles, whilst the posterior rectus sheath is made up of the other half of the internal oblique and transversus abdominis aponeuroses and the transversalis fascia.

Below the arcuate line, the anterior rectus sheath comprises the aponeuroses of the external oblique, internal oblique and tranversus abdominis muscles, whilst the posterior rectus sheath comprises only the transversalis fascia. Scarpa's fascia is a distinct layer separate from the rectus sheath.

41. Answers

A True
B True
C True
D False
E False

Sacculations, haustrations, the presence of three taeniae coli, appendices epiploicae, increased diameter and thicker wall all indicate large bowel. Both large and small bowel have longitudinal peristalsis and both have regions with and without a mesentery.

42. Answers

A True
B False
C True
D True
E False

Age incidence peaks for osteogenic sarcoma are 10–25 years and 40–60 years. Wide excision and chemotherapy is the standard treatment; amputation is only required in 20% of cases. It affects only 1% of patients with Paget's disease. It has a characteristic appearance on X-ray, showing a destructive lesion with surrounding new bone formation (sun-ray spicules), and there may be elevation of the surrounding periosteum (Codman's triangle).

43. Answers

A False
B False
C True
D False
E True

The second, third and fourth parts of the duodenum are all retroperitoneal. Most of the pancreas is retroperitoneal, except for the tip of the tail, which lies in the splenorenal ligament. The ascending and descending colon are retroperitoneal. The stomach, spleen, first part of the duodenum, transverse colon and sigmoid colon all have a mesentery.

44. Answers

A False
B True
C False
D False
E True

Renin converts angiotensinogen to angiotensin I. Angiotensin II is a powerful vasoconstrictor, which also stimulates the adrenal cortex to release aldosterone. Cortisol is not affected.

45. Answers

A True
B True
C True
D True
E True

46. Answers

A False
B True
C True
D False
E False

Carcinoma of the pancreas is more common in women (3:1) and more common in smokers. The peak incidence is in patients aged 60–80. It has an average 5-year survival rate of only 2–5%. Median survival after surgical resection is 18 months, and after palliative therapy only 5 months. In most cases the tumour is too far advanced for surgical resection, this being possible in only 8–25% of patients.

47. Answers

A True
B True
C False
D False
E False

Carcinoma of the oesophagus is 7 times more common in men. It is associated with Barrett's oesophagus, achalasia, corrosive strictures and Plummer–Vinson syndrome. In Asia 80% are squamous cell carcinomas, in the west 50%. Ivor–Lewis oesophagectomy is suitable for middle- and lower-third tumours. The 5-year survival rate is 5–6%.

48. Answers

A False
B True
C True
D False
E True

Thyroid, breast, bronchus, renal, prostate and haematological malignancies are the most common types to metastasize to bone. Osteosarcoma is a primary malignancy of bone but may metastasize to bony sites elsewhere.

49. Answers

A True
B True
C True
D False
E False

The incidence of melanoma is increasing (50% in the last decade). Superficial spreading lesions account for 70%, nodular melanomas 15% and acral lentiginous 10%, and the remaining 5% includes lentigo maligna and amelanotic melanomas. Breslow thickness, ulceration, site of the primary, presence of a vertical growth phase, sex, and the presence of lymphatic or visceral metastases affect prognosis. Melanomas on the trunk carry a worse prognosis than those on the limbs.

50. Answers

A False
B True
C False
D True
E False

Thyroid cancer is 3 times more common in women. It is more common in patients previously exposed to radiation and in those with pre-existing benign thyroid conditions (Hashimoto's disease and multinodular goitre). 70% are papillary, 16% are follicular, 6% are medullary, 7% are anaplastic and 1% are lymphomas. Papillary cancers carry the best prognosis and anaplastic cancers the worst. Medullary carcinomas of the thyroid form part of the MEN type 2A syndrome.

51. Answers

A True
B False
C True
D False
E True

Serum calcitonin is a useful marker for medullary cancers. The surgical treatment of thyroid cancer is total thyroidectomy, although small papillary tumours may be treated with lobectomy alone. Radioactive iodine can be used in the treatment of follicular carcinomas, advanced papillary carcinomas and metastatic disease. *Medullary* carcinomas may be associated with parathyroid adenomas and phaeochromocytomas – the MEN type 2A syndrome. Local invasion of the tumour into the recurrent laryngeal nerve will cause a hoarse voice.

52. Answers

A True
B False
C True
D False
E False

Lung cancer is the most common malignancy in western countries. 30% are squamous cell (best prognosis), 20% are small cell (worst prognosis) and 40% are adenocarcinomas (less related to smoking than other cell types). Pancoast tumours may invade the brachial plexus, causing C8/T1 syndrome.

53. Answers

A True
B True
C True
D True
E True

Other risk factors include air pollution, any form of tobacco smoke, coal and tar fumes, nickel, chromium, iron oxide, arsenic, and previous lung cancer.

54. Answers

A True
B False
C False
D True
E True

Most cancers arise in the peripheral zone. Bony metastases are common, but usually cause sclerotic lesions. All prostate cancers are adenocarcinomas, but with a varying degree of differentiation, which reflects aggressiveness. Other prostate disease may elevate PSA, but levels above 10–15 ng/ml suggest cancer.

55. Answers

A True
B True
C False
D False
E True

In western countries pancreatitis is most commonly due to either gallstones or alcohol. Iatrogenic causes include ERCP, drugs (thiazides, steroids and azathioprine) and surgery. Hypercalcaemia may cause pancreatitis, but pancreatitis usually causes a *hypo*calcaemia. Pancreatitis is usually managed by surgeons, but patients rarely need operative treatment for the condition – this is associated with a much poorer prognosis. Pancreatitis secondary to hyperlipidaemia is often more severe than gallstone or alcohol pancreatitis.

56. Answers

A False
B False
C True
D False
E True

Ranson's criteria give a score for each of the following:

On admission: age > 55; glucose > 11.2 mmol/l; WBC > 16; LDH > 350; AST > 250.

Within 24 hours: haematocrit fall > 10%; a rise in urea > 5 mg/l; calcium < 2.0 mmol/l; fluid sequestration > 6 litres; base excess > – 4; pO_2 < 8 kPa.

57. Answers

A True
B False
C False
D True
E False

Phaeochromocytoma is the 'tumour of 10%': 10% are malignant, 10% are bilateral, 10% are extra-adrenal (neck, thorax, kidney), 10% are familial, 10% occur in children, 10% are multiple. They may be detected be finding increased levels of VMA in the urine (urinary 5-HIAA goes up in carcinoid tumours). Phaeochromocytomas form part of the MEN type 2A and 2B syndromes.

58. Answers

A False
B True
C True
D False
E False

Metaplastic polyps are not premalignant. Peutz–Jeghers syndrome is the association between intestinal hamartomas and periorbital pigmentation. Polyps may bleed, leading to iron-deficiency anaemia. Villous adenomas are more prone to malignant transformation than tubulovillous adenomas, which are more prone to malignant transformation than tubular adenomas. Osler–Weber–Rendu syndrome is a familial syndrome characterized by multiple telangiectasia of the skin and of the oral, nasal and gastrointestinal mucous membranes.

59. Answers

A False
B False
C False
D False
E True

Familial adenosis polyposis is an autosomal dominant disease carried on the short arm of chromosome 5. The disease affects most patients in their 20s and 30s. Most patients undergo total colectomy with or without ileal pouch formation to prevent the development of bowel cancer. Gardner syndrome is the association between colonic polyps and widespread epidermoid cysts and osteomas.

60. Answers

A False
B False
C True
D False
E False

Approximately 5–10% of breast cancers are hereditary. Centrally located tumours are a relative indication for mastectomy. Recent overview studies have shown no benefit in giving tamoxifen in hormone receptor-negative tumours. Patients with small areas of DCIS do not need any axillary procedures. Radiotherapy is given after breast-conserving surgery to produce recurrence rates equivalent to mastectomy.

61. Answers

A True
B False
C False
D True
E True

H. pylori infection is thought to be the main initiating factor in peptic ulcerative disease. Due to the widespread use of H_2 antagonist and proton pump inhibitor medication, these patients now rarely present with surgical complications (perforation or bleeding). PUD is more common in developed countries and more common in smokers. The Zollinger–Ellison syndrome is a gastrin-secreting pancreatic tumour causing widespread peptic ulceration.

62. Answers

A False
B True
C True
D False
E False

H. pylori is a Gram-negative micro-aerophilic, spiral-shaped organism. It has been shown to increase gastric acid secretion sixfold. The organism contains urease, which splits urea into ammonia and carbon dioxide, thus *increasing* the pH locally, and protecting the organism from the acidic environment in the stomach. It is most commonly treated with '*triple* therapy': a proton pump inhibitor and a combination of two antibiotics.

63. Answers

A True
B False
C True
D True
E True

Aldosterone levels rise due to hypovolaemia stimulating renin release. Testosterone levels fall. Cortisol rises due to ACTH release. Noradrenaline and adrenaline both increase.

64. Answers

A True
B False
C True
D True
E False

Atherosclerotic plaques are within the intima and encroach on the media. They contain cellular and extracellular components as well as lipids and cholesterol. Thrombosis is usually triggered by plaque rupture, which exposes the very thrombogenic plaque contents to the circulating blood. Atherosclerosis of the distal aorta and common iliacs may lead to buttock claudication and impotence (Leriche syndrome). Atherosclerosis rarely affects the upper limb. The most common cause of upper limb ischaemia is thoracic outlet syndrome (compression of the subclavian artery).

65. Answers

A True
B True
C False
D True
E False

'Reducible' or modifiable risk factors include smoking, diabetes, hypertension, high cholesterol, obesity and physical inactivity. Male sex and positive family history are non-reducible risk factors. HRT was once thought to be protective against atherosclerosis, but recent evidence from the Heart and Estrogen/Progestin Replacement Study (HERS) suggests that there is no reduction in endpoint vascular disease in women taking HRT.

66. Answers

A False
B True
C True
D True
E True

Type A thoracic aortic dissections involve the ascending aorta and may involve any other part of the arch or descending aorta as well. Type B dissections only involve the descending aorta (i.e. distal to the left subclavian artery). Type A dissections have a better prognosis if managed surgically. Type B dissections are usually managed medically. Dissection of the coronary ostia will cause myocardial infarction with characteristic ECG changes.

67. Answers

A True
B False
C True
D False
E False

Predisposing factors for urinary calculi are increased concentration of solute in the urine (e.g. due to dehydration – common in busy surgeons!) and reduced solubility of solute in the urine (e.g. due to changes in urinary pH). The most common type are calcium oxalate stones (80%); 'triple phosphate' (magnesium, ammonium, calcium phosphate) stones comprise 15% of cases. Inflammatory bowel disease is a cause of hyperoxaluria that may precipitate as calcium oxalate stones. Prolonged irritation of the urothelium leads to squamous metaplasia, which may progress to *squamous cell carcinoma*. Most stones pass spontaneously, rarely requiring surgery.

68. Answers

A True
B False
C True
D True
E False

Gallstone formation is thought to be due to an imbalance of cholesterol and bile pigments. Excessive cholesterol (e.g. due to obesity) or reduced bile salt concentration (e.g. due to reduced enterohepatic circulation in Crohn's disease) leads to precipitation of cholesterol stones. Increased hepatic secretion of bilirubin (e.g. in haemolytic anaemias) leads to pigment stone formation. The majority of gallstones are 'mixed'. Neither viral hepatitis nor cirrhosis increase the risk of gallstone formation.

69. Answers

A True
B False
C False
D True
E False

Influenza virus is an RNA myxovirus, measles virus is an RNA paramyxovirus, and HIV is an RNA retrovirus.

70. Answers

A False
B True
C True
D False
E True

Iron deficiency causes a microcytic anaemia. Koilonychia is the development of brittle concave nails. Plummer–Vinson syndrome is the association of iron-deficiency anaemia with oesophageal web formation. Vitamin B_{12}- and folate-deficiency anaemia (megaloblastic) leads to painful swollen tongue. Iron deficiency may cause atrophy of tongue papillae. Menstruation makes iron deficiency more common in women.

71. Answers

A True
B False
C True
D True
E False

72. Answers

A False
B False
C False
D False
E False

Shaving disrupts deep skin flora and causes abrasions. Hair should be removed with clippers or depilatory cream immediately preop. MRSA-positive patients should be put at the end of the operating list because of the risk of cross-contamination. Steroids do impair wound healing, but should not be stopped as this may induce Addisonian crisis. In fact, supplementary IV hydrocortisone may need to be given to cover the stress of surgery.

73. Answers

A False
B True
C True
D False
E False

'Clean' wounds are incisions through non-inflammed tissue with no entry into GU/GI/respiratory tracts. 'Clean-contaminated' wounds are entry into a hollow viscus other than the colon with minimal contamination. 'Contaminated' wounds are entry into a hollow viscus with spillage of contents, entry into the colon, open fracture or animal bites. 'Dirty' wounds involve operating in the presence of gross pus, perforated viscus or peritonitis.

74. Answers

A False
B False
C False
D False
E False

Arterial blood pressure is proportional to cardiac output *multiplied* by systemic vascular resistance. Mean arterial pressure is approximately equal to the diastolic pressure plus one-third of the pulse pressure (systolic minus diastolic). The dichrotic notch corresponds to the *closing* of the aortic valve. The carotid bodies regulate respiration. The carotid sinus contains the baroreceptors. A fall in blood pressure is a late sign of hypovolaemia.

75. Answers

A False
B True
C False
D False
E False

The first heart sound corresponds to *closing* of the mitral and tricuspid valves; the second heart sound corresponds to closing of the aortic and pulmonary valves. Valves opening do not make a sound. The QRS complex is the depolarization of the ventricles that initiates ventricular systole. It is the opening of 'slow' *calcium* channels that causes the plateau phase of the cardiac action potential. The a-wave of the jugular venous waveform corresponds to atrial contraction. The A–V node *slowly* conducts the action potential from the atria to the ventricles, thus allowing a pause between atrial systole and ventricular systole.

76. Answers

A True
B False
C False
D False
E True

The anterior pituitary gland secretes prolactin, LH, FSH, TSH, growth hormone and ACTH. The posterior pituitary gland secretes oxytocin and ADH. Thyroxine is secreted by the thyroid gland. GnRH is released by the hypothalamus.

77. Answers

A False
B False
C True
D True
E True

Normal GFR is approximately 125 ml/min. 70% of sodium is reabsorbed in the proximal convoluted tubule. Sodium is actively pumped out of the thick ascending limb of the loop of Henle. This segment is impervious to water, and thus creates a sodium concentration gradient. ADH permits more water reabsoption in the collecting ducts, thus making the urine more concentrated.

78. Answers

A False
B True
C False
D False
E False

The vital capacity is equal to the inspiratory reserve volume added to the expiratory reserve volume *plus the tidal volume*. Vital capacity is easily measured using spirometry, but total lung capacity includes the residual volume, which is harder to measure. An FEV1/FVC ratio of *less* than 0.7 implies an *obstructive* lung defect; an FEV1/FVC ratio of *more* than 0.7 implies a *restrictive* lung defect. The residual volume is the amount of air that remains in the lungs at the end of maximal expiration. The dead space is the volume of the lungs/airway that does not partake in respiration.

79. Answers

A False
B True
C True
D True
E True

Haemoglobin consists of an Fe-containing porphyrin ring with *four* globin polypeptides. The oxygen dissociation curve has a sigmoid shape. The Bohr effect is a right shift of the dissociation curve by increased pCO_2, increased temperature, reduced pH or increased 2,3-DPG.

80. Answers

A False
B True
C True
D False
E True

Vitamin D is converted to 25-hydroxyvitamin D in the liver; this is then converted to 1,25-dihydroxyvitamin D (the active form) in the kidney. The final step is increased in the presence of PTH. Vitamin D can be obtained from the diet and also manufactured in the skin by the action of UV light on a cholesterol derivative. 1,25-Dihydroxyvitamin D increases calcium absorption from the intestine. Lack of vitamin D may lead to rickets in children or osteomalacia in adults.

81. Answers

A True
B True
C False
D False
E True

The average menstrual cycle lasts approximately 28 days. It is divided into the follicular phase (the end of which corresponds to ovulation) and the luteal phase (the end of which corresponds to menstruation). Ovulation is triggered by an LH surge. The corpus luteum secretes oestrogen and progesterone; the luteal phase therefore corresponds to higher levels of progesterone.

82. Answers

A False
B True
C True
D True
E False

The Golgi tendon apparatus is responsible for monitoring muscle tension; it sends inhibitory signals when stimulated, preventing excessive tension in the muscle/tendon that may lead to damage. The muscle spindle receptors monitor muscle stretch and are therefore responsible for the knee jerk reflex, which is a monosynaptic reflex. Acetylcholine acts on nicotinic receptors at the neuromuscular junction. Muscle contraction is calcium-dependent.

83. Answers

A True
B False
C False
D False
E True

Swimmer's view improves the view of the lower cervical vertebrae. Only the upper part of the vertebral body of T1 is required. The atlanto-odontoid gap is 2.5 mm in adults and 4 mm in children.

84. Answers

A False
B True
C False
D False
E True

The scalenus anterior muscle attaches superiorly to the anterior tubercles of the transverse processes of the C3–C7 vertebrae and inferiorly to the scalene tubercle of the 1st rib. The subclavian vein passes anteriorly to the muscle, whereas the subclavian artery and the brachial plexus pass posteriorly.

85. Answers

A True
B False
C False
D True
E True

The carotid artery lies in the carotid sheath, which is a layer of fascia anterior to the prevertebral layer of deep cervical fascia. The sympathetic chain lies behind the carotid sheath. The carotid sinus is a dilatation of the common carotid artery that contains baroreceptors. The internal carotid artery has no branches in the neck. The external carotid artery has 8 branches:

ascending pharyngeal
superior thyroid
lingual
facial
occipital
posterior auricular
superficial temporal
maxillary

(There is a mnemonic for these vessels, but unfortunately it is unprintable!)

86. Answers

A True
B False
C False
D False
E True

The thyroid gland lies within the pretracheal fascia, wrapped around the upper part of the trachea. It comprises two lobes, with a central isthmus at the level of the 2nd and 3rd tracheal rings. Its blood supply is from the superior thyroid artery (a branch of the external carotid artery) and the inferior thyroid artery (a branch of the thyrocervical trunk, which is a branch of the 1st part of the subclavian artery). 10% of people have a thyroid ima artery that arises from the arch of the aorta or occasionally the brachiocephalic artery and runs up the anterior surface of the trachea.

87. Answers

A False
B True
C True
D True
E False

Hyperacute rejection is antibody-mediated (cf. acute rejection, which is cell-mediated). It is due to preformed antibodies caused by previous blood transfusions, pregnancy and/or previous failed transplants. It is treated by removal of the transplant. Corticosteroids have a role in the treatment of acute rejection.

88. Answers

A False
B False
C False
D False
E True

The tibialis anterior, *extensor* digitorum longus and *extensor* hallucis longus all run in the anterior compartment. The lateral compartment of the leg is supplied by the superficial peroneal nerve; the deep peroneal nerve supplies the anterior compartment. Damage to the peroneal nerve causes foot drop; damage to the tibial nerve causes paralysis of the flexor muscles of the leg and intrinsic muscles of the sole of the foot, leading to an inability to plantarflex. The common peroneal nerve winds superficially around the neck of the fibular, where it is commonly damaged during fractures here.

89. Answers

A True
B True
C False
D True
E False

90. Answers

A False
B True
C True
D False
E True

The latissimus dorsi muscle is supplied by the thoracodorsal nerve, which arises from the posterior cord of the brachial plexus. It inserts into the floor of the bicipital groove of the humerus between the insertion of the pectoralis major and teres major muscles ('lady between two majors'). It derives its blood supply from the thoracodorsal artery, a branch of the subscapular artery, itself a branch of the second part of the subclavian artery.

Practice Paper 2: Answers

1. Answers

A True
B True
C False
D False
E True

Mycotic aneurysms develop when a vegetative endocarditis or an infected embolus lodges in the systemic circulation. Typical organisms are TB, *Salmonella* and *S. aureus.*

2. Answers

A False
B True
C False
D False
E True

Buerger's disease usually affects young (usually in their 30s) male smokers

3. Answers

A True
B False
C True
D True
E True

Dissecting aortic aneurysms are usually due to cystic medial necrosis (i.e. affecting the tunica media of the arterial wall). They usually start in the ascending aorta and may cause cardiac tamponade. Symptoms may be similar to an MI, although there are not usually the ECG changes unless the coronary ostia are involved.

4. Answers

A True
B True
C True
D True
E True

Technetium-99m scintigraphy and colour flow Doppler are helpful in showing the presence or absence blood flow in the testis and to differentiate from infective orchitis (increased vascularity). After 6 hours of ischaemia, the testis is less likely to survive – hence the indication for emergency surgery. A bell-clapper testis is a high-lying, horizontally positioned testicle.

5. Answers

A False
B True
C True
D True
E True

Pseudo-obstruction is initially treated conservatively by making the patient nil-by-mouth, inserting an NG tube and giving IV fluids. There is usually a predisposing cause, such as renal failure, significant chronic airways disease, spinal or pelvic fractures, or general debility. These causes should be treated where possible. If the condition persists, colonoscopic (or sigmoidoscopic) decompression may help. Caecostomy may be considered if these other measures fail, or else the bowel may (rarely) perforate.

6. Answers

A True
B True
C True
D False
E False

The dilutional hyponatraemia and haemodilution occur because of absorption of the irrigation fluid used (which does not contain calcium).

7. Answers

A True
B True
C False
D True
E True

Inguinal hernias are much more common in boys and premature infants. They should be repaired once diagnosed due to the risk of strangulation – unlike umbilical hernias, which often resolve by the age of 5 years. As there is no posterior wall weakness, a herniotomy is all that is required.

8. Answers

A True
B False
C False
D False
E True

Hepatitis B, C and D are spread by the blood/sex route. Hepatitis A and E are spread by the faecal–oral route.

9. Answers

A True
B True
C True
D True
E True

Rhabdomyolysis is a syndrome caused by the release of muscle cell contents (especially myoglobin) into the plasma following skeletal muscle injury. Known causes are ischaemic (e.g. vascular injury or compartment syndrome), muscle injury (seizures, burns, electric shocks or immobilization), infection (*E. coli* or *Salmonella*) and diabetic ketoacidosis.

10. Answers

A False
B True
C True
D False
E True

Acute mediastinitis is a very dangerous condition, resulting in marked systemic disturbance and sometimes cardiovascular collapse. It is caused by a full-thickness rent in the oesophagus (e.g. Boerhaave's rupture or instrumentation), by penetrating trauma or as a complication of cardiac surgery. Characteristic chest X-ray features, such as mediastinal widening or pneumomediastinum, are seen.

11. Answers

A True
B False
C True
D True
E False

Burns result in fluid loss from the circulation due to increased capillary permeability. This causes oedema and a drop in plasma volume leading to a reduced preload and hence a reduced cardiac output. Metabolic rate may double. Lung damage from inhalation causes bronchospasm, mucus production and decreased lung compliance. This may lead to ARDS. Escharotomy is required for circumferential chest burns to improve expansion and ventilation.

12. Answers

A True
B False
C False
D False
E True

The mnemonic 'SITS' will help you remember the structures that make up the rotator cuff: subscapularis, infraspinatus, supraspinatus and teres minor.

13. Answers

A True
B True
C True
D True
E True

14. Answers

A False
B True
C True
D False
E True

The blood supply comes from distal to proximal in the talus, scaphoid and head of the femur, predisposing them to AVN. Note that a fracture of the neck of the femur causes AVN in the head of the femur.

15. Answers

A True
B True
C True
D True
E True

Air may enter the bloodstream when the saphenous vein is opened prior to stripping, and also during intravenous transfusion. CO_2 may enter the bloodstream via laparoscopic surgery. Nitrogen bubbles may appear after decompression following deep-sea diving.

16. Answers

A True
B True
C True
D False
E False

The lower third is now the commonest site for carcinoma; the upper third is the least common site. The thoracic oesophagus lies posterior to the recurrent laryngeal nerve; the trachea lies anterior.

17. Answers

A False
B False
C True
D False
E True

The femoral triangle is bounded by the inguinal ligament, the medial border of the sartorius and the medial border of the adductor longus. It contains the adductor longus, pectinius and iliopsoas in its floor. It contains the femoral nerve and vessels as well as the anterior branch of the obturator nerve.

18. Answers

A True
B False
C False
D True
E True

IRV + TV = IC; ERV + RV = FRC; IRV + TV + ERV = VC; VC + RV = TLC; IRV + TV + ERV + RV = TLC

19. Answers

A True
B True
C True
D True
E True

Trash foot and ischaemic colitis result from embolization. The prosthetic graft may become infected. Paraplegia results from injury to the spinal vessels. Incisional hernia may follow any laparotomy.

20. Answers

A False
B True
C True
D False
E False

Testicular torsion does not produce a groin lump. Psoas abscesses classically point in the groin. Lymphoma is a differential for any lymphadenopathy. Saphena varix is only present when the patient is standing. A spigelian hernia is situated along the linea semilunaris of the abdominal wall.

21. Answers

A True
B False
C False
D False
E True

Silk and nylon are non-absorbable. Dexon and Vicryl are absorbed within several weeks, whereas PDS is absorbed in 6 months.

22. Answers

A True
B True
C False
D False
E True

DIC results in consumption of platelets and clotting factors. Massive transfusion dilutes the number of platelets and may require a separate platelet transfusion. Aspirin affects platelet function, not number. Warfarin has no effect on platelets. Heparin causes heparin-induced thrombocytopenia in a small number of patients.

23. Answers

A True
B True
C False
D False
E False

Beer's law indicates that the concentration of a solute can be determined by light absorption. Carbon monoxide produces carboxyhaemoglobin in the blood, which has a brighter-red appearance, affecting pulse oximetry readings. Nail polish underestimates the oxygen saturation. Oximetry uses two light wavelengths.

24. Answers

A True
B True
C False
D False
E True

In grade III shock, 30–40% of blood has been lost. Heart rate is usually over 120 bpm, systolic blood pressure is reduced, whereas diastolic pressure may increase due to vasoconstriction – hence a narrowed pulse pressure. Urine output falls to 20–30 ml/h. Respiratory rate rises to >20. The patient is also confused.

25. Answers

A True
B False
C False
D True
E False

The flexor digitorum profundus (FDP) inserts into the distal phalynx of the digits. The flexor digitorum superficialis (FDS) inserts into the middle phalynx of the digits. The lumbricals arise from the FDP tendon, run across the radial aspect of the corresponding metacarpal–phalangeal joint (MCPJ) and insert into the dorsal expansion of the corresponding digit. All intrinsic muscles of the hand are supplied by the ulnar nerve apart from the 'LOAF' muscles, which are supplied by the median nerve: lateral 2 lumbricals, opponens pollicis, abductor pollicis brevis and flexor pollicis brevis.

26. Answers

A True
B True
C False
D True
E True

Death following recent surgery or a drug error must be reported to the coroner. The death following chest drain in a patient who is not acutely unwell suggests that the death may be due to the chest drain itself. Mastoid bruising suggests a basal skull fracture; an NG tube is contraindicated in this situation as it may enter the cranial cavity.

27. Answers

A True
B False
C False
D False
E True

Wasting of the thenar eminence and the 1st and 2nd lumbricals are characteristics of median nerve palsy. Radial nerve injury causes a weakness of wrist extension.

28. Answers

A False
B False
C True
D False
E False

Renin release is stimulated by a drop in blood pressure and salt depletion. Propranolol inhibits renin release. Angiotensin II inhibits renin release as a negative-feedback mechanism. Increased plasma K^+ also inhibits renin release.

29. Answers

A False
B False
C True
D True
E False

Redcurrant jelly stools occur with intussusception. Necrotizing enterocolitis is a disease of the newborn. The aetiology involves bowel ischaemia followed by bowel wall invasion by gas-producing bacteria.

30. Answers

A False
B True
C True
D True
E True

31. Answers

A True
B True
C True
D True
E True

32. Answers

A True
B False
C True
D True
E False

Diverticulitis typically causes left iliac fossa pain. Curtis–Fitz-Hugh syndrome results from *Chlamydia* infection and produces bow-stringing around the liver. Charcot's triad is a feature of ascending cholangitis. Beck's triad is a feature of cardiac tamponade.

33. Answers

A True
B True
C True
D False
E True

Since *Pneumococcus* is the commonest organism in otitis media, amoxicillin is a good choice of antibiotic. For painful, bulging eardrums, myringotomy may be performed to release the pus. Perforation of the eardrum relieves the pain. Epileptic fits may occur if a cerebral abscess forms.

34. Answers

A True
B True
C False
D False
E False

Radiotherapy reduces spinal cord compression by reducing soft tissue swelling initially. Chemotherapy may cause nausea and vomiting in patients. Sclerosis takes longer to occur.

35. Answers

A False
B True
C False
D False
E False

The following are the signs of volume overload: tachycardia, raised JVP, 3rd heart sound, lung crepitations, oedema, tachypnoea.

36. Answers

A False
B True
C False
D False
E True

Breast cancer affects 1 in 9 women in the UK. The Nottingham Prognostic Index is used. Incidence continues to increase with age.

37. Answers

A False
B False
C False
D True
E False

Lignocaine is less effective in inflamed areas due to the local acidosis, which shifts the drug towards the ionized form, which is less effective. Increasing the concentration speeds up the onset of action, but still gives the same overall anaesthetic effect. The maximal dose is 3 mg/kg, or 7 mg/kg with adrenaline. Adrenaline should not be injected into peripheries, such as digits, tip of nose and ear lobes.

38. Answers

A True
B True
C False
D True
E True

Patients with a GCS of 12 are still conscious and can maintain their airway. GCS of less than 8 is an indication for intubation. This alone is, therefore, not an indication for a definitive airway.

39. Answers

A True
B True
C True
D False
E False

The uterus begins to rise out of the pelvis after the 12th week of pregnancy, and is therefore somewhat protected from abdominal injuries before this time. Because of the increased plasma volume, signs of hypovolaemia may be later than usual. The patient should be transported on her left side to avoid undue IVC compression, which reduces cardiac output and aggravates the shock.

40. Answers

A False
B True
C True
D True
E False

At autopsy, about 10% of men in their 50s can be shown to have small latent tumours, this number increasing to 70% of men in their 80s. However, it is estimated that only 10% of men over 65 will develop clinically significant prostate cancer. An increased incidence in American blacks has been reported.

If a 1 cm nodule is detected, it is cancer about 50% of the time. Prostatic biopsy is readily performed with little morbidity and is often required to confirm the diagnosis. Serum PSA is used to aid in the early detection of prostate cancer. PSA is elevated in 68% of men with cancer, but 33% of men with benign enlargement of the gland also have an enlarged PSA. Serum prostatic acid phosphatase is not specific for prostatic cancer, although a significant elevation is usually associated with metastatic disease. Serum acid phosphatase, however, has been generally replaced as a tumour marker by the immunoassay for PSA. PSA is also an extremely sensitive tumour marker for recurrences after surgery because serum levels should be undetectable if patients are tumour-free.

41. Answers

A True
B True
C True
D True
E True

Renal failure occurs because of graft rejection. Renal artery stenosis and ureteric obstruction occur because of anastomotic strictures. Other complications of renal transplantation include infections, glomerulonephritis, coronary artery disease, cerebrovascular disease, malignancy, avascular necrosis, obesity, Cushing syndrome and cataracts. Many of these are due to the steroids used.

42. Answers

A False
B True
C True
D False
E False

Indications for thoracotomy are initial drainage of >1000 ml blood, cardiac tamponade and cardiorespiratory arrest. Tension pneumothorax and empyema are treated by chest drainage.

43. Answers

A True
B False
C False
D True
E True

The anterior boundary is the free edge of the lesser omentum containing the portal triad (the portal vein posteriorly, the hepatic artery medially and the common bile duct laterally). The Pringle manoeuvre is where the portal vein and hepatic artery are pinched between the index finger in the epiploic foramen and the thumb anteriorly. This is useful to gain control of a bleeding liver laceration. The posterior boundary is the peritoneum over the inferior vena cava. The inferior boundary is the peritoneum over the first part of the duodenum. The superior boundary is the caudate process of the liver.

44. Answers

A False
B True
C True
D False
E True

Paget's disease of the breast is associated with cancer in 90% of cases and is an indication for surgery. It may be diagnosed by cytology of a nipple scrape, which shows pagetoid cells. Paget's disease of the bone is associated with normal calcium and elevated alkaline phosphatase.

45. Answers

A True
B False
C False
D True
E True

Cortisol actually enhances gluconeogenesis. Peak levels occur at 8.00 am.

46. Answers

A True
B False
C True
D False
E False

Urobilinogens are colourless, whereas urobilins (and stercobilins) are coloured. A fraction of urobilinogen is reabsorbed as part of the enterohepatic circulation of bile salts. β-Glucuronidases deconjugate bilirubin in the intestine. Conjugated bilirubin is excreted via an active transport system, as it is against a diffusion gradient.

47. Answers

A False
B True
C False
D True
E False

Only 2% of potassium is found extracellularly. Potassium is largely an intracellular ion. Hyperkalaemia stimulates aldosterone release, since this hormone causes the kidney to retain sodium and lose potassium. If the Na^+/K^+ pump is impaired, the intracellular potassium leaks out into the extracellular compartment and causes hyperkalaemia.

48. Answers

A False
B False
C True
D False
E True

Phosphate is the principal buffer in urine. Hydrogen ions are secreted into the renal tubules in exchange for sodium ions. Ammonia (NH_3), not ammonium ions (NH_4^+), can cross the membranes of renal tubular cells. The hydrogen ion concentration is proportional to the CO_2 in the blood ($CO_2 + H_2O = H^+ + HCO_3^-$).

49. Answers

A True
B False
C True
D True
E False

The rectus abdominis muscle crosses the costal margin as it originates from the costal cartilages of the 5th, 6th and 7th ribs. It usually has three tendinous intersections: at the xiphisternum, at the umbilicus and one in-between. It has a dual blood supply: the superior epigastric artery (a terminal branch of the internal mammary artery) and the inferior epigastric artery (a branch of the external iliac artery). The transverse rectus abdominis muscle (TRAM) flap is used in breast reconstruction. The nerve supply is segmental from anterior rami of the inferior six thoracic and first lumbar nerves.

50. Answers

A True
B True
C False
D True
E True

There is protein catabolism initially.

51. Answers

A True
B True
C False
D True
E True

The palatine tonsil lies posterior to the palatoglossal arch. The glossopharyngeal nerve supplies the tonsil.

52. Answers

A False
B True
C True
D True
E True

Most regard 65–70 years as the upper limit for day surgery.

53. Answers

A True
B False
C True
D True
E True

Graduated compression stockings should not be given to patients with significant peripheral vascular disease.

54. Answers

A True
B False
C True
D False
E True

H. pylori infection is present in 30% of the adult population, but increases with age. It may be detected by the presence of labelled carbon dioxide in the breath following administration of labelled urea (urease breath test). Triple therapy can be expected to cure 70–90% of cases. *H. pylori* is now thought to be an aetiological factor in gastric cancer.

55. Answers

A False
B True
C True
D True
E True

BMI may be used: this is weight divided by height squared. Measuring urinary urea gives an estimate of nitrogen balance, which is an important way of assessing a patient's nutrition. Bioelectrical impedence gives an estimate of lean body mass. Serum transferrin levels reflects nutritional states more accurately than albumin.

56. Answers

A True
B False
C True
D True
E False

Elemental diets contain amino acids and oligopeptides as their source of nitrogen. Polymeric diets contain whole protein, complex carbohydrates and fat, as well as vitamins and trace elements. Jejunostomies reduce the risk of pulmonary aspiration compared with gastric feeding.

57. Answers

A True
B True
C False
D True
E True

Hypercapnia may occur as a result of the respiratory failure component.

58. Answers

A True
B True
C True
D True
E False

CO_2 embolism is a rare complication. Bradycardia often occurs during establishment of the pneumoperitoneum. CO_2 absorption may produce an acidosis. The pneumoperitoneum may reduce venous return to the heart – hence falling cardiac output.

59. Answers

A True
B False
C True
D False
E True

Cyclosporin may cause nephrotoxicity, hepatotoxicity, tremors, convulsions, hirsutism, rashes, gingival hypertrophy, haemolytic anaemia, hypertension and malignant changes.

60. Answers

A False
B True
C False
D True
E False

Dextrose saline is 4% dextrose and 0.18% saline. Normal saline is 0.9% saline, which contains 155 mmol/l sodium and chloride ions. 5% dextrose provides negligible calorific value.

61. Answers

A True
B True
C True
D True
E True

62. Answers

A False
B True
C False
D False
E False

With the exception of DIC, the others are all associated with a normal thrombin time.

63. Answers

A True
B True
C True
D True
E False

Citrate ions are contained within the transfusion bags. These viruses are not screened for. Prolonged bleeding arises as a result of low platelets and clotting factors. Hypersplenism does not occur.

64. Answers

A True
B True
C True
D True
E False

ITP does not cause Raynaud's phenomenon, whereas thrombocytosis does.

65. Answers

A True
B False
C False
D False
E False

The LSV is formed by the union of the dorsal vein of the great toe and the dorsal venous arch and ascends anterior to the medial maleolus. It runs superficial to the deep fascia of the leg (crural fascia) just behind the palpable posterior medial border of the tibia. It passes a hand's breadth behind the medial border of the patella and then joins the femoral vein at the saphenofemoral junction, 2 cm below and medial to the femoral pulse, by piercing the fascia lata. Although some evidence suggests that arterial grafts are superior to venous grafts, long-term data are missing. LSV grafts are still widely used in CABG surgery.

66. Answers

A True
B True
C True
D True
E True

67. Answers

A False
B False
C True
D True
E True

Rectal prolapse has an increased incidence in the first year of life and then again in old age. It is 20 times commoner in women in old age, but of equal incidence before this.

68. Answers

A True
B False
C False
D False
E False

Pringle's manoeuvre is used to stop bleeding from the liver. Charcot's triad consists of jaundice, right upper quadrant pain and pyrexia. ERCP is the commonest reason for air in the biliary tree. 75–90% of gallstones are mixed stones, whereas only 10% are cholesterol stones. Pigment stones and calcium carbonate stones are the least common.

69. Answers

A False
B True
C True
D False
E False

The platysma, facial artery and vein, and the cervical branch of the facial nerve lie superficial to the gland. The hypoglossal and lingual nerves and digastric muscle lie deep to the gland.

70. Answers

A False
B True
C False
D True
E True

The external branch of the superior laryngeal nerve is at risk during thyroidectomy as it lies near the superior poles of the gland. The ilioinguinal nerve lies within the inguinal canal, which is not opened in the low approach to a femoral hernia. Damage to the sural nerve is a common cause for litigation in varicose vein surgery. The intercostobrachial nerve is frequently damaged during axillary clearances.

71. Answers

A True
B False
C False
D True
E False

Urachal remnant tumours are usually adenocarcinomas. The male-to-female ratio is approximately 3 : 1. T2 tumours invade the muscle but are not palpable after resection.

72. Answers

A False
B True
C True
D True
E False

The strap muscles are supplied by the ansa cervicalis. The sternohyoid lies in front, the sternothyroid and thyrohyoid lie behind, and the omohyoid laterally. The inferior belly of the omohyoid attaches to the superior border of the scapular, it passes through a fascial sling attached to the medial clavicle and then inserts into the inferior border of the hyoid bone. The anterior belly of the digastric is supplied by a branch of the mandibular division of the trigeminal nerve, the posterior belly is supplied by the facial nerve. The mylohyoid is supplied by the same nerve that supplies the anterior belly of the digastric.

73. Answers

A True
B False
C False
D True
E True

Treatment of head injury aims to minimize secondary brain injury. Hyperventilation may be helpful, since it reduces the $p\text{CO}_2$, which reduces intracranial pressure. Normal withdrawal scores 4 on the GCS motor response section.

74. Answers

A True
B True
C False
D False
E False

Infections and anastomotic dehiscences are both most common around day 5 postoperatively. Pyrexia > 41°C is almost always non-infectious; causes include malignant hyperpyrexia, heat stroke, hypothalamic disorders and drug reactions. DVT often causes a low-grade pyrexia, which classically occurs at day 10.

75. Answers

A False
B False
C True
D False
E False

The most common ECG abnormality is a sinus tachycardia. S1Q3T3 is the pattern to be recognized. Although it can present at any time postoperatively, it classically presents at day 10. The most accurate investigation is a pulmonary angiogram.

76. Answers

A True
B False
C False
D True
E True

Central cord syndrome is usually seen after a hyperextension injury. It is characterized by a greater loss of motor power in the upper limbs than in the lower limbs.

77. Answers

A True
B True
C False
D False
E True

Indications for cardiopulmonary bypass are repair of intracardiac defects, replacement of cardiac valves, CABG, supradiaphragmatic aortic surgery, heart/lung transplantation, cardiac support and hypothermia.

78. Answers

A True
B False
C True
D True
E False

Combination chemotherapy should ideally contain drugs that have different mechanisms of action, that should all be active against the tumour when used alone, and that should have minimally overlapping toxicities. Neoadjuvant chemotherapy refers to chemotherapy given prior to surgery rather than following surgery.

79. Answers

A False
B True
C False
D False
E True

Only about 10% of patients walk again following an above-knee amputation. Scars should specifically not transmit pressure, as this can impair healing and cause pain. The PAM aid should be applied early at 5–7 days postoperatively.

80. Answers

A True
B False
C True
D True
E True

2 cm capsule lacerations of the spleen are classified as a grade II injury (Moore's classification). Grades I–III should ideally be treated conservatively initially and followed-up by regular CT scanning. Grades IV and V require emergency splenectomy.

81. Answers

A False
B False
C False
D True
E False

Loss of axonal continuity is known as axonotmesis (e.g. crushing injuries), whereas neurotmesis refers to section of the nerve. The axon grows at 1 mm/day following injury. It is the distal axon that undergoes Wallerian degeneration. Delayed repair (3–4 weeks) is preferable in contaminated wounds.

82. Answers

A True
B False
C True
D False
E True

The pH of uniting fractures starts to increase after the 10th day (alkaline tide). Although hyperparathyroidism causes bone demineralization and pathological fractures, there is no evidence that it impairs the healing of fractures.

83. Answers

A True
B False
C False
D True
E True

Cholinergic impulses occur in the parasympathetic nervous system, as opposed to adrenergic impulses in the sympathetic nervous system. Parasympathetic stimulation causes detrusor muscle and gallbladder contraction. It also causes increased intestinal mobility and erection. Vagal stimulation causes decreased atrial contractility.

84. Answers

A False
B True
C True
D True
E False

The brain receives 15% of the cardiac output (approximately 750 ml/min in a 70 kg adult). The intracranial pressure rises with the intracranial volume in a nonlinear (exponential) relationship.

85. Answers

A True
B False
C False
D True
E False

Cullen sign (periumbilical bruising) indicates intraperitoneal blood, as with severe haemorrhagic pancreatitis. In spinal cord injury there is disruption of sympathetic output, and hence bradycardia, urinary retention, hypotension and priapism.

86. Answers

A True
B True
C True
D True
E True

The effects of endotoxic shock are due to the endotoxin (a lipopolysaccharide from the bacterial cell wall) stimulating the release of cytokines that influence thermoregulation and metabolic responses. The subsequent vasodilation causes hypotension (hence shock) and warm peripheries. The other complications (ARDS, oedema and haemorrhage) arise as a consequence of MODS.

87. Answers

A False
B True
C True
D True
E False

Anterior shoulder dislocation is much more common than posterior dislocation. The arm is held in the abduction position and there is flattening of the shoulder contour.

88. Answers

A False
B True
C False
D False
E False

Cells are sensitive to ionizing radiation during M and G_2 phases. During G_1 the cells are active, synthesizing RNA and proteins. The duration of the cell cycle is constant in malignant tumours, but not in normal tissues. The cells of solid tumours pass through the cell cycle at different phases.

89. Answers

A False
B True
C True
D False
E True

Gut flora usually cause abscesses of the appendix. Finger pulp infection may be caused by *S. aureus* via a penetrating wound. Ischiorectal abscesses usually contain faecal flora.

90. Answers

A False
B True
C False
D True
E True

$CD8^+$ cells recognize antigen in conjunction with MHC class I molecules. Cell-mediated (type IV) hypersensitivity reactions take 12–24 hours to develop.

Practice Paper 3: Answers

Theme: Blood transfusion

1. **A** – Patients with blood group A have anti-B antibodies and therefore cannot receive any group B blood.
2. **D** – Patients with blood group B have anti-A antibodies and therefore cannot receive any group A blood. (Patients with group AB blood have no antibodies and therefore can receive any blood.)
3. **E** – The Rhesus antigen is less important than the ABO. However, a young woman who is Rhesus D-negative and is exposed to the Rhesus D antigen (via transfusion or childbirth) will develop antibodies that may attack a subsequent Rhesus D-positive fetus. To prevent this, the mother is given anti-D immunoglobulin at the time of the birth, which reduces her own immune response.
4. **F** – Transfusion is usually only necessary when the Hb drops to below 8 g/dl or in symptomatic patients.
5. **D** – Patients with blood group O have both anti-A and anti-B antibodies and therefore can only receive group O blood.

Theme: Breast disease

6. **A** – Fibroadenomas are the commonest type of breast lump in young women. They are usually very mobile – hence the name breast mice.
7. **F** – Blood-stained discharge, nipple inversion, hard fixed lumps, skin dimpling (peau d'orange) and skin inflammation/ulceration are all suspicious signs of malignant breast disease.
8. **B** – Fat necrosis can be difficult to distinguish clinically from malignancy. Here the core biopsy indicates that the lesion is benign: B1, normal; B2, benign breast tissue; B3, equivocal, probably benign; B4, suspicious, probably malignant; B5, malignant.
9. **G** – Duct ectasia is dilatation of the larger ducts containing stagnant or infected fluid. Green discharge is characteristic.
10. **F** – This woman has metastatic breast cancer. Cytology is reported in a similar manner to core biopsy: C1, inadequate; C2, benign; C3, equivocal, probably benign; C4, suspicious, probably malignant; C5, malignant.

Theme: Groin lumps

11. **B** – Varicocoeles are very common (10% of the population have them). They are more common on the left side, as the left testicular vein drains into the left renal vein at 90°, whereas the right testicular vein drains directly into the IVC at a more acute angle (acting like a valve). They characteristically disappear on lying and feel like a bag of worms.
12. **H** – Epididymo-orchitis is an infection of the epidymis and testis. Patients present with a painful, swollen testicle that is easily confused with testicular torsion, but the onset is usually more insidious.

13. **D** – Any lump in the scrotum that the examining hand cannot get above has to be assumed to arise from the inguinal canal. In this age group indirect hernias are much more common than direct hernias, and are due to a patent processus vaginalis. This is more common on the right.
14. **E** – A hydrocoele is a collection of fluid within the tunica vaginalis that transilluminates. The testis lies within the fluid collection. A hydrocoele of the cord is felt as a discrete cyst along the cord that again transilluminates.
15. **A** – Any solid lump in the scrotum must be assumed to be a cancer until proven otherwise. Testicular cancers are often associated with a small hydrocoele.

Theme: Neck lumps

16. **G** – Cystic hygromas are not true cysts but rather lymphangiomas. They usually present early in childhood but smaller ones may not be noticed till later. They characteristically transilluminate brilliantly.
17. **A** – Any lump that moves on swallowing must be attached to the larynx or trachea. Most commonly, these are thyroid swellings.
18. **B** – The submandibular gland especially is prone to form stones. These may partially obstruct Wharton's duct, leading to pain and swelling in the gland.
19. **I** – A midline lesion that rises on protruding the tongue is a thyroglossal cyst.
20. **D** – Epidermal (or sebaceous) cysts are common on the face, neck, scalp and trunk. They lie within the skin and usually have a characteristic punctum.

Theme: Thyroid disease

21. **E** – Most thyroid cancers are 'cold nodules', i.e. they do not secrete T_4. This women has hyperthyroidism secondary to a T_4-secreting adenoma.
22. **C** – Multinodular goitre is a common finding. It is due to the development of simple non-toxic colloid nodules and cysts. Patients are euthyroid. Large or retrosternal goitres may compress the trachea or oesophagus.
23. **A** – Graves' disease is an autoimmune condition. Circulating antibodies bind to and stimulate the TSH receptors of the thyroid gland, leading to hyperplasia and marked hyperthyroidism.
24. **B** – Hashimoto's disease is another autoimmune condition. There is diffuse lymphocytic invasion of the thyroid gland, leading to swelling, tenderness and progressive hypothyroidism. It may be associated with other autoimmune conditions such as pernicious anaemia.
25. **G** – Endemic goitre is now rare in the UK. It is due to iodine deficiency and leads to diffuse hyperplasia of the thyroid gland. It is common in landlocked and mountainous regions that are deprived of fish and other seafood rich in iodine.

Theme: Thyroid cancer

26. **C** – Medullary carcinoma is an uncommon tumour of the medullary C cells (which secrete calcitonin). It may form part of the MEN type 2 syndrome (associated with phaeochromocytoma and parathyroid adenomas).

27/ 29. **D** – Papillary carcinoma is the most common type of thyroid malignancy and tends to affect younger age groups. The sex ratio (F : M) is 3 : 1. It is more common in patients exposed to radiation. It metastasizes early to lymph nodes. There is a 90% 10-year survival rate.

28. **A** – Anaplastic thyroid cancers affect an older age group. They are locally aggressive and metastasize early. They have a poor prognosis.

30. **E** – Thyroid lymphomas account for 2% of thyroid malignancies and often arise with Hashimoto's disease. Most are non-Hodgkin lymphomas. There is a good prognosis with radiotherapy.

Note: Follicular thyroid cancers are impossible to differentiate from benign follicular adenomas on FNA. The peak incidence is at age 40–50. The female-to-male ratio is 3 : 1. Metastases are late and usually via the bloodstream to lungs and bone. There is an 85% 10-year survival rate.

Theme: Hepatobiliary disease

31. **B** – This woman has a history typical of cholecystitis. Ultrasound will confirm the presence of gallstones and will show gallbladder wall thickening and fluid. A plain abdominal X-ray is unnecessary as only 10% of gallstones are radio-opaque.

32. **C** – This man has alcoholic pancreatitis. The temperatures and WBC suggest development of pancreatic necrosis/abscess. Contrast CT will show how much pancreas is necrotic (does not take up contrast) or the presence of collections/pseudocysts.

33. **A** – This woman has symptoms and signs of bowel obstruction. The gallstones may be a coincidence or may be the cause through the very rare diagnosis of gallstone ileus. Plain X-ray will show dilated loops of bowel.

34. **D** – This man has obstructive jaundice due to a stone in the CBD. ERCP is indicated to further delineate the anatomy and also remove the stone if possible.

35. **F** – This woman has carcinoma of the head of the pancreas and obstructive jaundice. If ERCP is unsuccessful at stenting the CBD then external drainage via PTC is indicated to relieve the jaundice and prevent further renal damage.

Theme: Hip fractures

36/ 39. **A** – A dynamic hip screw is the treatment of choice for extracapsular fractures. This can be performed under a spinal anaesthetic if the patient has other comorbidity preventing a general anaesthetic. This should be attempted in all patients who were previously mobile, as the prolonged bed rest required for treatment by traction predisposes to thromboembolic disease and chest infections.

37. **E** – In young patients the head of the femur should be preserved if possible, as prostheses have a limited lifespan. Two or three cannulated screws can be used to fix the head.
38. **B** – In the older patient the treatment of choice for intracapsular fracture is a hemi-arthroplasty (uncemented in the very elderly or patients with severe comorbidity due to the increased risk of fat embolism). However, patients with pre-existing arthritis may benefit from having a total hip replacement, as the prosthetic head would not glide smoothly in a diseased acetabulum.
40. **G** – An intramedullary hip screw combines an intramedullary nail for fixing a shaft of femur fracture with a sliding screw extending into the head of the femur to stabilize the neck.

Theme: Flexor tendon injuries

41. **B** – Zone 2.
42. **A** – Zone 1.
43. **E** – Zone 5.
44. **B** – Zone 2.
45. **D** – Zone 4.

- Zone 1 is distal to the insertion of the FDS tendon (i.e. only the FDP tendon). The surface marking is half way between the PIPJ crease and the DIPJ joint crease.
- Zone 2 is between the A1 pulley and the insertion of the FDS tendon (corresponding to the area where the FDS and FDP tendons run in the flexor sheath). The surface markings are the distal palmar crease to the middle of the middle phalynx.
- Zone 3 is between the flexor retinaculum and the A1 pulley (FDS and FDP are unsheathed).
- Zone 4 is within the carpal tunnel (under the flexor retinaculum).
- Zone 5 is proximal to the flexor retinaculum.

Theme: Salter–Harris classification of fractures

46. **D** – Type 4.
47. **E** – Type 5.
48. **B** – Type 2.
49. **A** – Type 1.
50. **C** – Type 3.
51. **B** – Type 2.

- Type 1 is a fracture through the epiphyseal plate.
- Type 2 is a fracture through the epiphyseal plate and including some of the metaphysis.
- Type 3 is a fracture through the epiphyseal plate and through the epiphysis into the joint.
- Type 4 is a fracture through the epiphysis, epiphyseal plate and metaphysis.
- Type 5 is a crush fracture of the epiphyseal plate, and is often missed initially.

Theme: Lower limb injuries

52. **H** – The tibial nerve supplies all the muscles in the posterior compartments of the lower leg and can be damaged as it runs behind the tibia during knee surgery.
53. **A** – The extensor hallucis longus muscle is supplied by the L5 myotome, and the 1st web space is the L5 dermatome.
54. **F** – The deep peroneal nerve is at risk of damage as it winds around the neck of the fibula. It supplies the muscles of the anterior compartment of the lower leg and sensation to the 1st web space.
55. **D** – The sciatic nerve is the most important structure to protect during hip surgery. It supplies all the muscles below the knee and all the sensation to the lower leg, except for the medial side, which is supplied by the saphenous nerve.
56. **J** – The sural nerve runs close to the short saphenous vein and supplies sensation to the outside of the foot.

Theme: Upper limb injuries

57. **D** – The radial nerve is at risk of damage as it winds around the posterior surface of the midshaft of the humerus. It supplies all the extensors of the wrist.
58. **H** – Avulsion of the C5/C6 nerve roots results in Erb's palsy (waiter's tip position). It is also common following birth trauma.
59. **B** – This child has a supracondylar fracture of the humerus. This injury commonly damages the median nerve, thus causing numbness in the thumb (as well as index and middle fingers).
60. **F** – The anterior interosseous nerve arises from the median nerve and runs on the volar surface of the interosseous membrane. It supplies the flexor pollicis longus, the lateral half of the flexor digitorum profundus and the pronator quadratus.
61. **G** – The axillary nerve is at risk of injury in anterior shoulder dislocation as it is relatively fixed at its origin (the posterior cord of the brachial plexus) and its insertion into the deltoid muscle. It is also at risk from humeral neck fractures, as it passes through the quadrangular space. The axillary nerve supplies the teres minor and deltoid and sensation to the 'regimental badge' area.

Theme: Blood gases

62. **D** – The pH is raised; therefore this is an alkalosis. The CO_2 is reduced; therefore this is a respiratory alkalosis. There is no compensation. An example is hyperventilation.
63. **A** – The pH is low; therefore this is an acidosis. The CO_2 is also low; therefore this is a metabolic acidosis. The negative base excess confirms this. The low CO_2 is attempting to compensate for the acidosis. An example is sepsis.
64. **H** – The pH is slightly raised and the CO_2 is low; therefore this is a respiratory alkalosis. However, the pH is not very low and the base excess is raised. This is a result of the kidneys compensating for the alkalosis. An example is acclimatization to altitude.

Theme: Rectal bleeding in children

65. **F** – Painful anal fissures are the result of constipation and lead to a vicious cycle where the child refuses to open their bowels, thus worsening the situation. Haemorrhoids are not common in children of this age.
66. **B** – Necrotizing enterocolitis is most common in sick or premature neonates. Plain X-ray shows intramural gas.
67. **D** – Meckel's diverticulae may cause rectal bleeding as they often contain heterotopic gastric mucosa. This shows up with a technetium-99m scan.
68. **E** – The symptoms suggest either IBD or an infective cause. The duration suggests IBD.
69. **C** – This history is classic of colic. Intussusception commonly occurs between 6 and 9 months. The 'redcurrant jelly' stool is caused by the blood mixed with mucus. A sausage-shaped mass may be palpable in the abdomen.

Theme: ATLS classification of haemorrhage

70. **B** – Class II.
71. **C** – Class III.
72. **A** – Class I.
73. **D** – Class IV.
74. **B** – Class II.

- Class I haemorrhage is when less than 15% of the circulating volume is lost (total volume is approximately 5 litres in a 70 kg man). There may be a mild tachycardia but no other cardiovascular changes.
- Class II haemorrhage is when 15–30% of the circulating volume is lost (approximately 750 ml–1.5 litres). There is tachycardia and tachypnoea, and the pulse pressure may narrow (due to a rise in diastolic pressure secondary to catecholamine release), but there is no drop in systolic pressure. Urine output is mildly affected.
- Class III haemorrhage is when 30–40% of the circulating volume is lost (approximately 2 litres in a 70 kg man). This is defined as the lowest volume loss to produce a reliable drop in systolic blood pressure. There is tachycardia, tachypnoea, hypotension, reduced mental function and oliguria.
- Class IV haemorrhage is when more than 40% of the circulating volume is lost. This is immediately life-threatening. There is marked tachycardia, tachypnoea, very narrow pulse pressure, hypotension, possibly unconsciousness and anuria.

Theme: Burns

75. **B** – 9%.
76. **C** – 18%.
77. **B** – 9%.
78. **B** – 9%.
79. **A** – 1%.

- The 'rule of nines' is a method for calculating the surface area involved in burns. This divides the body into 11 units of 9% and the remaining 1% for the perineum. Each arm is 9%, each leg is 2×9%, the front of the torso is 2×9%, the back of the torso is 2×9% and the head is the remaining 9%. Another way of estimating surface area is to use the patient's palm, which corresponds to about 1%.

Theme: Urological symptoms

80. **F** – Nocturia, terminal dribbling, hesitancy, poor stream, urgency and frequency are all symptoms of bladder outflow obstruction. A PSA of 4.5 ng/ml is just above the upper limit of normal for his age, thus making the diagnosis of BPH more likely than prostate cancer.
81. **E** – Urethral strictures are common after urethritis.
82. **G** – Urinary tract infections can present with many symptoms in the elderly. They are more common in the presence of a foreign body (e.g. a catheter).
83. **H** – Ureteric calculi classically cause back, flank and loin pain, which may radiate to the testicles. Vomiting is a common symptom.
84. **B** – Bladder calculi often sit at the neck of the bladder; therefore they may lead to outlet obstruction and urinary retention. Sharp stones may burst the catheter balloon.

Theme: Peripheral vascular disease

85. **K** – Leriche syndrome is a combination of erectile dysfunction, buttock and thigh claudication with or without muscle wasting. It is due to distal aortic stenosis. Aorto–biiliac bypass would restore blood to the pelvic vessels as well as the femorals.
86. **I** – An axillo–bifemoral bypass is an extra-anatomical bypass, and can even be performed under local anaesthetic for the high-risk patient.
87. **C** – Below-knee amputation is always preferable to above-knee amputation if possible. Radiolucency of the bones under an infected ulcer suggests probable osteomyelitis. These ulcers will never heal without improving the arterial inflow to the limb. However, such extensive arterial disease with no run-off makes vascular reconstruction impossible.
88. **F** – Acute limb ischaemia (which may be on a background of chronic ischaemia) suggests an embolism, especially in the presence of atrial fibrillation. Embolectomy is the treatment of choice.
89. **E** – Such a small segment of stenosis is amenable to percutaneous angioplasty or stenting.
90. **H** – Extensive areas of stenosis make stenting impractical. Bypass grafting is more appropriate, but only if the distal run-off is adequate.

Theme: Prostate cancer

91. **F** – Small, well-differentiated cancers have been shown to have a high 10-year survival rate with no treatment. In older men they can therefore be kept under observation.
92. **A** – Large studies have shown benefit from prostatectomy over other forms of treatment for poorly differentiated tumours with no metastatic disease. There is, however, a higher incidence of side-effects (e.g. incontinence, impotence and rectal injury). Brachytherapy is another option in these patients, but is now thought to be less effective for larger tumours.
93. **E** – Hormonal modification is the treatment of choice for advanced disease. Options include orchidectomy, oestrogens, LHRH analogues and anti-androgens.
94. **B** – Radiotherapy is useful to relieve the pain of bony metastases.

Theme: Jaundice

95. **F** – Courvoisier's law states that in the presence of jaundice a palpable gallbladder is more likely to be due to malignancy than gallstones. Stones cause chronic inflammation leading to a fibrosed gall bladder that cannot dilate. Cholangiocarcinoma is much rarer than carcinoma of the pancreas.
96. **C** – This woman has classic obstructive jaundice. The most likely cause is a stone in the CBD, although this is not always seen on ultrasound.
97. **A** – Unconjugated bilirubin implies a prehepatic cause of jaundice. In a patient with fever from an area where *Plasmodium falciparum* is endemic a diagnosis of malaria should be suspected.
98. **E** – Mirizzi syndrome is obstructive jaundice caused by external compression of the common hepatic duct by a gallstone in the gallbladder. This woman has acute cholecystitis. The upper limit of normal for the CBD is 10 mm diameter. An alternative diagnosis in a patient with right upper quadrant pain, fever and jaundice (Charcot's triad) is ascending cholangitis.
99. **B** – The ALT is grossly raised compared with the alkaline phosphatase, making a hepatocellular cause of jaundice most likely (e.g. viral hepatitis).
100. **H** – Sclerosing cholangitis is associated with ulcerative colitis in 70% of cases. There is a characteristic beading of the ducts on ERCP.

Theme: The paediatric abdomen

101. **A** – Meckel's diverticulae are relatively common (2% of the population) and may contain heterotopic gastric mucosa that may lead to ulceration and bleeding. They may also form the lead point for an intussusception.
102. **E** – Pyloric stenosis is more common in firstborn boys. It presents with projectile vomiting leading to a hypochloraemic alkalosis. The child is usually hungry following vomiting. A mass may be palpable in the epigastrium.
103. **H** – The incidence of duodenal atresia is 1 in 6000 and is more common in patients with Down syndrome. The double-bubble sign is diagnostic.

104. **G** – Malrotation is where the gut fails to form the correct anatomical position. The duodeno–jejunal junction lies to the right and the caecum lies in the left upper quadrant. A volvulus may occur, as the root of the mesentry is narrower. There is not usually abdominal distention, as the level of obstruction is high. There may be PR bleeding, indicating bowel ischaemia.

105. **C** – Intussusception is reported in 1 in 500 children. It is most common between 6 and 9 months. Most are ileocolic. There may be the characteristic redcurrant jelly stool.

Theme: Abdominal pain

106. **B** – Pyelonephritis usually presents with fever and loin pain. It is usually the result of an ascending UTI.

107. **G** – A hypernephroma or renal cell carcinoma is the commonest malignancy of the kidneys. It may also present as a pyrexia of unknown origin, anaemia or polycythaemia. Polycystic kidneys are more likely to present earlier and are bilateral.

108. **H** – The history of collapse, tachycardia and hypotension are suspicious of AAA. The pain may be felt in the abdomen, back or flank. The amylase may be raised due to the close position of the pancreas over the front of the abdominal aorta.

109. **K** – This woman has generalized peritonitis. The history of arthritis should alert you to the use of NSAIDs or steroids, which predispose to peptic ulcerative disease. The amylase is often raised after a perforated DU. Levels over 1000 iu/l are diagnostic of pancreatitis.

110. **J** – Appendicitis can be a difficult diagnosis to make. The symptoms here suggest a retrocoecal or pelvic appendix. Irritation of the neighbouring bladder can lead to urinary symptoms and signs.

Theme: Gastrointestinal investigations

111. **C** – The most likely diagnosis is peptic ulcer disease, but an OGD is necessary to exclude gastric carcinoma and to take biopsies for the CLO test (*Helicobacter pylori*).

112. **C** – This man is haemodynamically compromised. Despite the bleeding per rectum, the most likely source of such torrential bleeding is an upper GI source. Immediate OGD is indicated.

113. **B** – These symptoms sound like biliary colic. Ultrasound is a quick, non-invasive investigation that is usually very reliable. If this is normal, proceed to OGD.

114. **A** – Haemorrhoids are the most likely causes of his symptoms. Proctoscopy can diagnose and treat the condition (with banding).

115. **E** – This is a life-threatening upper GI bleed. If OGD is unsuccessful at stopping the bleeding then laparotomy is indicated. However, her previous surgery would make laparotomy slow and dangerous (multiple adhesions). Angiogram and embolization of the bleeding vessel is probably her best chance.

116. **D** – If sigmoidoscopy is normal then a colonoscopy is indicated. This can treat as well as diagnose the cause (e.g. AV malformation or polyp).

Theme: Upper gastrointestinal surgery

117/ 121. **I** – Whipple's procedure or pancreatico–duodenectomy is appropriate for periampullary tumours (pancreatic head tumours, low cholangiocarcinomas and duodenal tumours) without extensive local or distal spread. It is a major operation, with a mortality rate of 5–10%. Even with surgery, the 5-year survival rate is around 20%. The procedure involves resecting the distal stomach, the head, body and uncinate process of the pancreas, the duodenum, the common bile duct, and the gallbladder, and then attaching all the ends together.

118. **K** – This man has gastric outlet obstruction secondary to an unresectable gastric cancer. The priority here is to relieve symptoms. The simplest way is to bypass the tumour.

119. **C** – Signet ring cells are characteristic of the diffuse type of gastric adenocarcinoma. Malignant ulcers tend to have raised edges. As the tumour is high on the wall, a distal gastrectomy is not possible. A total gastrectomy with clearance of the local lymph nodes is indicated (R1 or R2).

120. **M** – Malignant ulcers of the duodenum are extremely rare. Much more common are peptic ulcers. If left, they may perforate into the peritoneal cavity or erode into the nearby vessels (e.g. gastroduodenal artery), causing torrential haemorrhage. This patient has had an unsuccessful trial of medical treatment. Surgical treatment involves dividing the parasympathetic nerve supply to the stomach, thus stopping acid production. Unfortunately, this also paralyses the stomach, slowing gastric emptying. For this reason, a pyloroplasty is also performed.

122. **L** – An unresectable tumour of the head of the pancreas is best treated by alleviating the symptoms. A triple-bypass procedure involves bringing up a loop of jejunum with a side-to-side anastomosis gastro–jejunostomy (to relieve duodenal obstruction), a cholecysto–jejunostomy (to relieve the biliary obstruction) and a side-to-side jejuno–jejunostomy to divert food away from the biliary tree.

Theme: Colorectal surgery

123. **B** – Tumours of the caecum and ascending colon are beast treated by right hemicolectomy and primary anastomosis of the terminal ileum to the transverse colon.

124. **H** – In the patient with obstruction and therefore dilated bowel, resection and primary anastomosis is unwise, as the risk of anastomosis breakdown is high. Hartmann's procedure is far safer. This involves resecting the sigmoid colon, and bringing the proximal end to the surface as an end-colostomy. The rectal stump is closed.

125. **L** – Low-rectal tumours are best treated with an abdominoperineal resection. This involves excising the rectum and anal canal and bringing out an end-colostomy. High-rectal tumours can be treated with an anterior resection.

126. **F** – Transverse colostomy is rarely carried out. Splenic flexure tumours are best treated with an extended left hemicolectomy.

127. **J** – This man has familial adenomatous polyposis coli. This is an autosomal dominant condition caused by a mutation on the short arm of chromosome 5. Affected patients develop many benign adenomatous polyps. If left, the progression to malignant transformation is inevitable. By removing all the colonic mucosa, the risk of cancer is eliminated. Panproctocolectomy with ileal pouch and ileoanal anastomosis is the treatment of choice.

Theme: Skin disease

128. **F** – Seborrhoeic keratoses are very common. They tend to occur in older patients in areas that are hard to reach when washing (e.g. the back). They may be mistaken for melanomas. They are usually multiple, and have a lighter brown pigment and a characteristic waxy, warty appearance. They can be picked from the skin, leaving a few bleeding capillaries.

129. **C** – BCCs are common and tend to occur around the face. They start as a nodule with a pearly appearance and surface telangectasia, but may progress to form an ulcer (rodent). They do not metastasize but are locally invasive.

130. **E** – This is a classic SCC. They tend to occur in sun-exposed areas. They metastasize to local lymph nodes.

131. **B** – The incidence of melanoma is increasing. It may occur de novo or in an existing mole. Suspicious features include darker pigmentation, asymmetrical lesions, rapid growth, ulceration or crusting, bleeding, itching, a halo, and satellite lesions.

132. **H** – This is a histiocytoma or dermatofibroma. About 20% are thought to arise in insect bites.

Theme: Diarrhoea

133. **D** – Appendicitis may cause diarrhoea. The abdominal tenderness and the short history of symptoms suggest this diagnosis.

134. **J** – Weight loss and obstructive jaundice must raise a suspicion of pancreatic cancer. The steatorrhoea is secondary to the lack of bile salts and thus reduced fat absorption.

135. **I** – Blind-loop syndrome is where stasis in a long afferent loop of bowel leads to bacterial overgrowth. This leads to impaired digestion and absorption of food. Vitamin deficiency (e.g. B_{12}) may occur.

136. **E** – Amoebic dysentery or amoebic colitis is caused by a protozoon parasite called *Entamoeba histolytica*. It is endemic in many developing countries. Less than 5% of carriers develop symptoms, which are caused by the organism invading the bowel wall. It may progress to toxic megacolon and liver abscesses.

137. **H** – Chronic alcoholism is a risk factor for chronic pancreatitis. Steatorrhoea develops because of reduced pancreatic exocrine secretions of lipase, leading to malabsorption of fats.

Theme: Carcinogens

138. F – Aflatoxin is a mycotoxin from *Aspergillus flavus*.
139. **C** – β-Naphthylamine is an aromatic amine used in the rubber and dye industry. It is converted in the liver to an active carcinogen, which is then concentrated in the urine.
140. **D** – UV light is the most important risk factor for the development of malignant melanomas, BCCs and SCCs.
141. **G** – Thyroid carcinoma, certain bone tumours and leukaemias are all increased in incidence in patients exposed to ionizing radiation.
142. **B** – Asbestos is now banned from the building industry because of the link to mesothelioma. It also predisposes to other types of lung cancer.
143. **A** – Squamous cell carcinoma of the scrotum was common in chimney sweeps in the 19th century.

Theme: Viral carcinogens

144. **H** – Human immunodeficiency virus.
145. **B** – Hepatitis B virus.
146. **D** – Epstein–Barr virus.
147. **G** – HTLV-I.
148. **E** – Human papillomavirus.
149. **D** – Epstein–Barr virus.
150. **D** – Epstein–Barr virus.

Practice Paper 4: Answers

Theme: Tumour markers

1. **B** – Alpha-fetoprotein.
2. **G** – Thyroglobulin.
3. **C** – CA 19-9.
4. **B** – Alpha-fetoprotein.
5. **F** – Calcitonin.
6. **E** – CA 125.

Theme: Mass in the right iliac fossa (RIF)

7. **A** – The fact that it is a health check suggests that he is well. The scar and mobile mass suggest that he has had a pelvic renal transplant.
8. **C** – Tiredness, weight loss and age suggest malignancy. The mass in the RIF suggests caecal cancer as the most likely cause.
9. **F** – His nationality, classical symptoms and anaemia suggest TB.
10. **G** – The age, RIF pain and fever suggest appendicitis. This has been partly treated with antibiotics, resulting in an appendix mass.
11. **B** – Some symptoms suggest either TB or lymphoma (night sweats, weight loss, fever). The itching and alcohol-induced pain suggest lymphoma.
12. **E** – A classical presentation. The contrast X-ray is pathognomonic.

Theme: Haematuria

13. **F** – Sudden onset of severe flank pain with haematuria suggests ureteric colic.
14. **A** – Age and classical symptoms suggest UTI.
15. **E** – Backache and X-rays suggest secondaries. In view of the nocturia and blood in urine, prostate cancer is most likely.
16. **B** – The CXR suggests cannonball metastases, which are associated with renal adenocarcinoma. The diagnosis is supported by the history.
17. **C** – Tyre factory workers have a higher risk of transitional cell carcinoma. The history and urine are consistent with the diagnosis.
18. **D** – Although prostate cancer is a possibility, benign growth is more common and therefore more likely.

Theme: Bone pain

19. **A** – The history suggests prostatic cancer with bony metastases.
20. **H** – The young age, white cell count, ESR and pyrexia suggest infection.
21. **C** – Pepperpot skull, anaemia and raised ESR all suggest myeloma.
22. **B** – The age, site of swelling and X-ray suggest osteosarcoma.
23. **D** – Abdominal and bone pain combined with X-rays suggest the diagnosis. Blood tests for PTH and calcium will confirm this.
24. **G** – The X-ray changes, increased alkaline phosphatase and limb deformity suggest the diagnosis.

Theme: Acid/Base Balance

25. **A** – There will be a lactic acidosis.
26. **D** – She will be hypoxic and thus hyperventilate, lowering the pCO_2.
27. **C** – This neuromuscular disease may cause hypoventilation due to paralysis of the respiratory muscles.
28. **B** – The mineralocorticoid excess results in a hypokalaemia and loss of hydrogen ions via the kidney, which results in alkalosis.
29. **A** – The fistula will predominantly lose bicarbonate, hence leading to acidosis.
30. **D** – She is likely to be hyperventilating – hence the faint feeling. This will bring about a respiratory alkalosis as CO_2 is removed from the lungs.

Theme: Blood constituents and their replacement

31. **E** – This patient has reasonable haemoglobin and platelet levels and is still bleeding. The large transfusion suggests that he/she is deficient of clotting factors – hence the need for FFP.
32. **B** – He appears to be haemodynamically stable, yet anaemic. There is no need for whole blood.
33. **G** – Cryoprecipitate is indicated for clotting factor replacement in von Willebrand's disease and haemophilias.
34. **H** – Although platelets are indicated for severe thrombocytopenia, the cause in this case is immune thrombocytopenia, which is best treated with immunoglobulin in the first instance. If the platelet count fell to dangerously much lower levels, platelets might also need to be given.
35. **A** – He has severe shock (stage III or IV). He is obviously losing blood at a fast rate given the 10-minute history. Whole blood would be preferable here due to its volume. An alternative would have been packed red cells with crystalloid, but the latter is not listed.
36. **D** – This is a dangerously low platelet count, which requires urgent replacement therapy.

Theme: Skin ulcers

37. **F** – Inflammatory bowel disease is a known association of pyoderma gangrenosum. The history of the ulcer is typical.
38. **A** – The features are typical of a venous ulcer with surrounding lipodermatosclerosis.
39. **H** – The history suggests that the wound became infected from organisms possibly originating from the sea. Coupled with the fact that she is young and presumably otherwise fit, the most likely diagnosis is a tropical ulcer. The organisms are usually spirochaetes and fusiform bacteria.
40. **C** – The history is typical of a squamous carcinoma developing in a chronic venous leg ulcer.
41. **E** – The fact that a relatively young man with both legs is in a wheelchair suggests a neurological condition. He has good blood supply and no evidence of venous disease. This combination makes neuropathic ulcer the most likely. He has had pressure on his heel from the wheelchair, but could not feel any discomfort.
42. **B** – A classic description of rest pain and foot ulcers in a male smoker.

Theme: Principles of cancer treatment

43. **C** – This cancer is not amenable to primary surgery. She needs neo-adjuvant chemotherapy followed by subsequent mastectomy.
44. **E** – Radiotherapy is the usual treatment, with a good outcome as squamous cell tumours are highly radiosensitive.
45. **B** – The histology and symptoms indicate Hodgkin lymphoma.
46. **F** – She now has metastatic breast cancer that persists despite two previous courses of chemotherapy. Hormonal therapy will not be of use in view of the negative ER and PR status. However, the monoclonal antibody trastuzumab (Herceptin) is of proven benefit in this situation.
47. **D** – He has metastatic prostate cancer. At this stage, it is best treated with drugs such as goserelin (Zoladex) (LHRH analogues).
48. **A** – Surgical excision is usually all that is required. An alternative treatment is radiotherapy, but as it is difficult for the patient to get to the hospital regularly, excision is simpler.

Theme: Treatment of vascular disease

49. **G** – He requires an elective aortic aneurysm repair with a graft.
50. **D** – This stenosis does not meet the 70% cut-off whereby a carotid endarterectomy would be offered. She should be medically managed and observed.
51. **C** – He is a candidate for intervention in view of the rest pain and quality of life. The only suitable procedure is a bypass from the common femoral artery to the distal vessels (fem-distal bypass). Vein grafts give better results than synthetic grafts in this situation.
52. **E** – The history and signs strongly suggest an embolus in the SFA, just after the bifurcation of the CFA. The predisposing cause is AF. She has a good chance of full recovery in view of the short history.
53. **A** – This type of lesion has a good outcome following angioplasty.
54. **B** – An extra-anatomical bypass, such as an axillo–bifemoral bypass, is a common solution to this difficult problem. Synthetic grafts are still required, in order to avoid kinking, although infection is still a risk.

Theme: Endocrine tumours

55. **G** – The X-ray features suggest hyperparathyroidism. Parathyroid adenoma is the most common cause. Parathyroid hyperplasia is rarer.
56. **D** – A classical presentation of carcinoid syndrome.
57. **E** – She has a high calcium and PTH, which indicates primary hyperparathyroidism. The bilateral milky nipple discharge in the absence of pregnancy suggests hyperprolactinaemia, although the prolactin level is awaited. The MEN type I syndrome includes parathyroid adenomas, pituitary adenomas and pancreatic cell tumours.
58. **C** – The symptoms are due to excessive serum levels of catecholamines, which are metabolized to VMA and excreted via the kidneys.
59. **F** – The elevated PTH and calcitonin suggest hyperparathyroidism and medullary thyroid cancer respectively. The past history of adrenalectomy raises the additional possibility of a phaeochromocytoma. These three conditions are recognized as the MEN type 2 syndrome.
60. **A** – It is actually unusual to see four hot spots in this condition. The scan is often negative. The diagnosis is usually made at operation and confirmed with frozen sections and subsequent histology.

Theme: Gastrointestinal haemorrhage

61. **F** – Colonoscopy is the best investigation for lower GI bleeding. In addition, it may be therapeutic if polyps are found.
62. **A** – The history, examination and X-rays suggest large-bowel obstruction. The history of age, recent hip surgery and airways disease combined with the lack of pain and bowel sounds suggest that this is a pseudo-obstruction rather than a mechanical obstruction, necessitating a contrast enema for diagnosis. The haemorrhoids and fresh blood are probably unimportant.
63. **E** – The most likely diagnosis is a bleeding peptic ulcer (duodenal or gastric), which may be diagnosed and treated via upper GI endoscopy.
64. **B** – The history of aortic stenosis raises the possibility of angiodysplasia of the right colon, which is a well-recognized association. She appears to be actively bleeding in view of the haemodynamic instability. Selective angiography would be useful in confirming the diagnosis and enabling subsequent embolization of the abnormal vessels, once the patient has been resuscitated.
65. **C** – Since there does not appear to be an upper or lower GI cause for the bleeding, a barium meal and follow-through enable the small bowel to be assessed. The lip pigmentation raises the possibility of Peutz–Jeghers syndrome, which is associated with benign polyps of the small intestine.

Theme: Pancreatic and hepatobiliary disease

66. **C** – Chronic severe pain, diabetes, malabsorption and the CT changes are characteristic. Biopsy is often needed to exclude carcinoma of the pancreas.

67. **J** – Her recent surgery is likely to have been for gallstones. The jaundice and dilated CBD suggest a retained CBD stone after surgery. However, she also has a fever and elevated white cell count, making ascending cholangitis the more likely development.

68. **B** – The inflammation of the gallbladder (acute cholecystitis) is causing the adjacent bile ducts to be obstructed either by direct pressure or due to inflammation of the duct walls. This may happen with a short cystic duct.

69. **E** – This is a classical presentation of a common disease.

70. **G** – The ERCP findings are characteristic of this rare conditions, which is associated with UC. It is radiologically indistinguishable from cholangiocarcinoma, which had been excluded in this patient.

71. **I** – A CT scan will usually confirm the diagnosis.

Theme: Anaesthetic techniques

72. **C** – He is unfit for a general anaesthetic, and epidural/spinal anaesthesia is effective and much safer in this situation.

73. **A** – As she is sensible and fit, a local anaesthetic is most suitable, although she may chose a general anaesthetic if she is anxious.

74. **D** – This requires muscle paralysis and may need bowel resection. GA is mandatory.

75. **C**

76. **B** – A Bier's block is usually performed.

Theme: Rectal bleeding

77. **I** – The pain was due to the ischaemic event to his colon (in the typical watershed area). He already has atherosclerosis of his coronaries, which makes the diagnosis more likely. The X-ray findings are typical.

78. **C**

79. **F** – This is the usual carcinoma found around the anus. It characteristically spreads via the lymphatics to the regional inguinal nodes.

80. **E** – The autosomal dominant gene is found on chromosome 5.

81. **B** – The fissure is seen with the 'sentinel pile' usually at the 6 or 12 o'clock position.

82. **H** – Classical history, examination and radiological findings. Biopsy confirms the diagnosis.

Theme: Breast cancer treatment

83. **A** – Tumours of this size require mastectomy and nodal clearance. In addition, lobular carcinomas are often even larger than their clinical and radiological size.
84. **E** – Radiotherapy is required after all wide excisions. Tamoxifen is required in ER-positive cancers. Chemotherapy is indicated in view of the positive nodes and relatively young age.
85. **H** – DCIS usually requires radiotherapy postoperatively unless it is low-grade and very small in size with wide margins, in which case no further treatment is required. Endocrine therapy is not routinely administered to patients with DCIS.
86. **I** – She will need chemotherapy at some stage in view of her young age, regardless of the exact final histology. Since it is grade 3, it is likely to respond well to chemotherapy. If given preoperatively, this may shrink the tumour enough to allow breast conservation.
87. **G** – She requires radiotherapy following breast conservation. She also needs hormonal therapy. Tamoxifen is not recommended for patients with a past history of DVT – hence the need for aromatase inhibitors.
88. **B** – Although she may also be offered mastectomy, wide excision gives the same long-term survival and is cosmetically more acceptable.

Theme: The Glasgow Coma Score

89. **D** – Eyes, Motor, Verbal = 2 + 4 + 1 = 7.
90. **C** – E + M + V = 1 + 3 + 2 = 6.
91. **H** – E + M + V = 3 + 5 + 4 = 12.
92. **A** – E + M + V = 1 + 1 + 1 = 3.
93. **B** – E + M + V = 1 + 2 + 1 = 4.
94. **I** – E + M + V = 3 + 6 + 4 = 13.

Theme: Preoperative investigations

95. **E** – The echocardiogram will assess her left ventricular function (ejection fraction), as well as the performance of her artificial valve.
96. **F** – He appears to have chronic airways disease. As he is undergoing a major procedure, he requires full respiratory assessment.
97. **A** – No indication for any routine tests.
98. **B** – She may be anaemic in view of her condition. In addition, she probably has pathology within her urinary tract, thus necessitating a basic assessment of her renal function.
99. **D** – In view of malignancy and her age, she needs the routine blood tests. Since she smokes, it is prudent to organize an ECG and CXR. The latter may also show metastases. A G&S is required, since a few patients occasionally require transfusion.
100. **C** – He should have these basic tests in case he has any subclinical cardiac or respiratory problems. The probability of these is increased since he is a smoker. No G&S is required with an MUA.

Theme: The acute abdomen

101. **B** – A typical presentation of severe acute pancreatitis with a positive Cullen sign.

102. **F** – The sudden onset of pain, known ischaemic heart disease, AF and lack of X-ray signs make this the most likely diagnosis. Arterial blood gases would show a metabolic acidosis and high lactate.

103. **A** – She appears to have a diverticular abscess, although this needs confirmation, ideally with an abdominal CT scan.

104. **G** – A chest X-ray would show air under the diaphragm.

105. **I** – Although no pulsatile mass was noted, he is obese. Still, he has three risk factors for atherosclerosis (smoking, obesity and diabetes) and has ischaemic heart disease. He is clearly shocked. In this situation, a ruptured aneurysm is the most likely diagnosis, which would have been seen on the CT scan.

106. **E** – An abdominal X-ray would confirm the clinical impression. The tenderness suggests imminent caecal perforation, necessitating urgent laparotomy.

Theme: Medicine and the law

107. **F**
108. **C**
109. **D**
110. **A**
111. **E**

Theme: The painful swollen knee

112. **C** – The anterior draw sign is diagnostic of this injury.

113. **F** – The obesity suggests joint overload. The findings are typical.

114. **D** – The findings suggest a medial collateral ligament injury.

115. **H** – Bucket handle tears and parrot's beak tears may be found with these injuries. The locking is due to a loose part of the cartilage getting stuck between the articular surfaces.

116. **B**

117. **G** – Lack of trauma limits the diagnosis to osteoarthritis, rheumatoid arthritis or gout. The short history and diagnostic fluid (negatively birefringent crystals) suggests gout.

Theme: Clinical examination tests

118. **C** – Tapping over the facial nerve results in twitching of the upper lip in hypocalcaemia.
119. **A** – The history is suggestive of a ruptured Achilles' tendon, which may be verified using this test.
120. **G** – Ortolani's modification of Barlow's test is positive in congenital dislocation of the hip.
121. **B** – Pain is elicited if the tibia is rotated on the femur with a torn meniscus.
122. **J** – This test may help decide if she has had a DVT (dorsiflexion of the foot causes pain), although a venous duplex scan is indicated.
123. **E** – This helps determine whether there is a patent ulnar artery supplying the palmar arch before harvesting the radial artery.

Theme: Anorectal surgery

124. **D** – Conservative management is the mainstay of treatment.
125. **C** – This is effective in approximately two-thirds of patients with anal fissures. For the remainder, a lateral sphincterotomy is required.
126. **E** – This is effective for grade II haemorrhoids.
127. **D** – The diagnosis is likely to be a thrombosed perianal varix (perianal haematoma). An alternative treatment is to incise the lesion under local anaesthesia and evacuate the small blood clot.
128. **F** – The only effective treatment for grade III haemorrhoids is haemorrhoidectomy.
129. **H** – Following GTN cream for anal fissures, surgery is the second-line treatment. Although anal stretch used to be performed, it had an unacceptably high minor incontinence rate.

Theme: Surgical sutures

130. **D**
131. **E**
132. **B** – A cosmetic result is desired.
133. **C**
134. **G** – Although a mass closure with loop PDS is an alternative, the chances of sound healing in the near future are low in this sick individual who has dehisced his previous sutures. Deep tension sutures are useful in this situation.
135. **A** – Fine sutures are required on the eyelids.

Theme: Visual field defects

136. **A**
137. **F**
138. **C**
139. **E**
140. **B**

Theme: Structures damaged during surgery

141. **G** – In the posterior approach to the hip, the sciatic nerve is at risk of damage. For this reason it is identified and then protected by swinging the short external rotator muscles over the top of it.

142. **A** – The ilioinguinal nerve is at risk of damage during any open inguinal hernia repairs. This leads to numbness of the base of the penis/labia majora/upper medial thigh and paralysis of the lower abdominal wall musculature.

143. **D** – The external laryngeal nerve is a branch of the superior laryngeal nerve and supplies the cricothyroid muscle. It runs close to the superior thyroid artery and is at risk of damage during ligation of this vessel. Damage to the external laryngeal nerve leads to weakness of the voice.

144. **J** – The marginal mandibular nerve (a branch of the facial nerve) runs just below the angle of the mandible and supplies the small muscle of facial expression that elevates the corner of the mouth. Incisions in this area must be placed two fingers' breadth below the angle of the mandible to avoid this structure.

145. **C** – The inferior parathyroid glands have a more variable anatomical position than the superior parathyroid glands but are commonly located near the inferior pole of the thyroid gland. The inferior thyroid artery and the recurrent laryngeal nerve lie close by. Damage to the recurrent laryngeal nerve may lead to a hoarse, croaking voice.

Theme: Lower limb trauma

146. **G** – A below-knee amputation is always preferable to an above-knee amputation. A Gustillo 3c fracture means that this is an open injury with extensive soft tissue loss, possibly with contamination and an associated vascular injury requiring repair. This leg is beyond salvage.

147. **A** – A spiral fracture of the lower tibia is likely to extend into the ankle joint, although it may not appear so on X-ray. IM nailing would open up this fracture and disrupt the ankle mortice. Skeletal traction can be used with good effect.

148. **B** – This fracture pattern can be treated in several different ways. IM nailing provides a rapid restoration of mobility and avoids the large incision and periosteal stripping needed for open plating of the tibia. An external fixator device (Ilizarov frame) can also be used, but is bulky and expensive, requires more skill to apply, and may lead to pin-site infections.

149. **C** – This fracture is ideally treated with cancellous screws to the medial maleolus and a plate with cortical screws to the fibula.

150. **D** – IM nails are hard to use in highly comminuted fractures and destroy the medullary marrow thought to be beneficial in fracture healing. In open fractures there is also the theoretical risk of prosthesis infection if there is a delay in achieving soft tissue cover. An external fixator device is the best way to achieve rapid bony stability. Care must be taken when orientating the pins not to compromise the vessels or the positioning of a freeflap.